The *Joy* of Dog Training

30 FUN, NO-FAIL LESSONS TO RAISE AND TRAIN A HAPPY, WELL-BEHAVED DOG

KYRA SUNDANCE

QUARRY

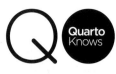

Inspiring | Educating | Creating | Entertaining

Brimming with creative inspiration, how-to projects, and useful information to enrich your everyday life, Quarto Knows is a favorite destination for those pursuing their interests and passions. Visit our site and dig deeper with our books into your area of interest: Quarto Creates, Quarto Cooks, Quarto Homes, Quarto Lives, Quarto Drives, Quarto Explores, Quarto Gifts, or Quarto Kids.

First Published in 2020 by Quarry Books, an imprint of The Quarto Group, 100 Cummings Center, Suite 265-D, Beverly, MA 01915, USA.
T (978) 282-9590 F (978) 283-2742 QuartoKnows.com

Quarry Books titles are also available at discount for retail, wholesale, promotional, and bulk purchase. For details, contact the Special Sales Manager by email at specialsales@quarto.com or by mail at The Quarto Group, Attn: Special Sales Manager, 100 Cummings Center, Suite 265-D, Beverly, MA 01915, USA.

10 9 8 7 6 5 4 3 2 1

ISBN: 978-1-63159-970-5

Digital edition published in 2020
eISBN: 978-1-63159-971-2

Library of Congress Cataloging-in-Publication Data

Names: Sundance, Kyra, author.
Title: The joy of dog training : 30 fun, no-fail lessons to raise and train a happy, well-behaved dog / Kyra Sundance.
Description: Beverly, MA : Quarry Books, 2020. | Includes index. | Summary:
    "The Joy of Dog Training is an engaging and interactive guide for training your dog by teaching them 30 fundamental tricks"– Provided by publisher.
Identifiers: LCCN 2020017148 | ISBN 9781631599705 (trade paperback) | ISBN 9781631599712 (ebook)
Subjects: LCSH: Dogs–Training.
Classification: LCC SF431 .S868 2020 | DDC 636.7/0835–dc23
LC record available at https://lccn.loc.gov/2020017148

Design: Kyra Sundance
Assistant Trainer: Claire Doré
Photography: Christian Arias

Printed in China

DoMoreWithYourDog.com

We aim not to suppress behavior and teach subservience, but rather to have a joyful relationship with a confident and happy dog who is motivated to do the right thing rather than fearful of making a mistake.

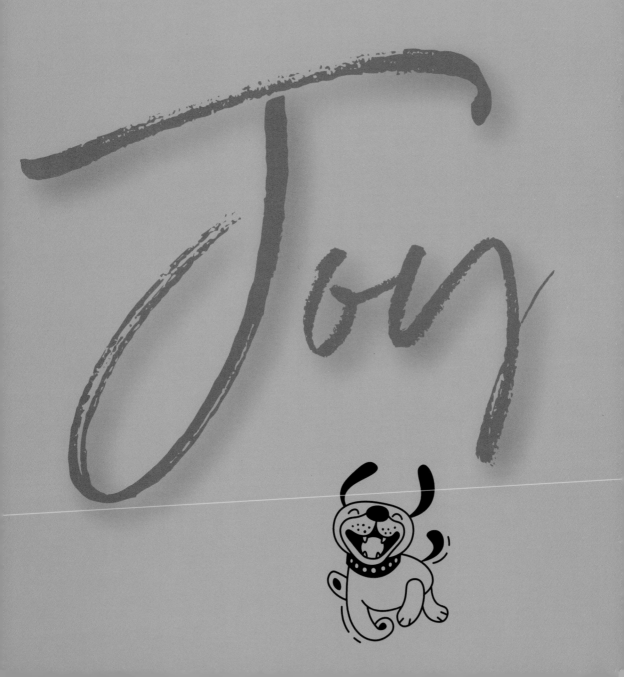

CONTENTS

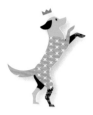

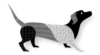

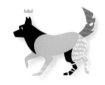

Introduction

As a professional stunt-dog performer, I've received top honors in dog sport competition and live entertainment shows. I believe in striving for and achieving lofty goals. But I also know that the enormous rewards I've gotten through training my dogs have come to me not through the end result of a goal met but rather through the connections I've built along the way, the lessons I've learned, and the joys of the experience. With this book I give you and your dog the tools to not only succeed in your training but to train humanely and joyfully.

Kickstart Your Enthusiasm!

Are you ready to break the monotony of routine and kickstart your enthusiasm for training? Then let's do it! This book will guide you through the process of training your dog in a way that's fun for you and for your dog. And because it's fun, it will be easy to stick with. This book will give you the knowledge and structured instruction to train successfully and without frustration. Concepts will be explained to you clearly, quickly, and simply. You will gain a new connection with your dog family member and a feeling of accomplishment at having learned a new skill and bettered the life of your dog.

Whether you are a **novice trainer** just starting out or an **intermediate trainer** who has been training intuitively and is now looking for academic structure, this book is for you. And for those of you **expert trainers** . . . this book might be a chance to side-step the quest for excellence and reclaim your joy!

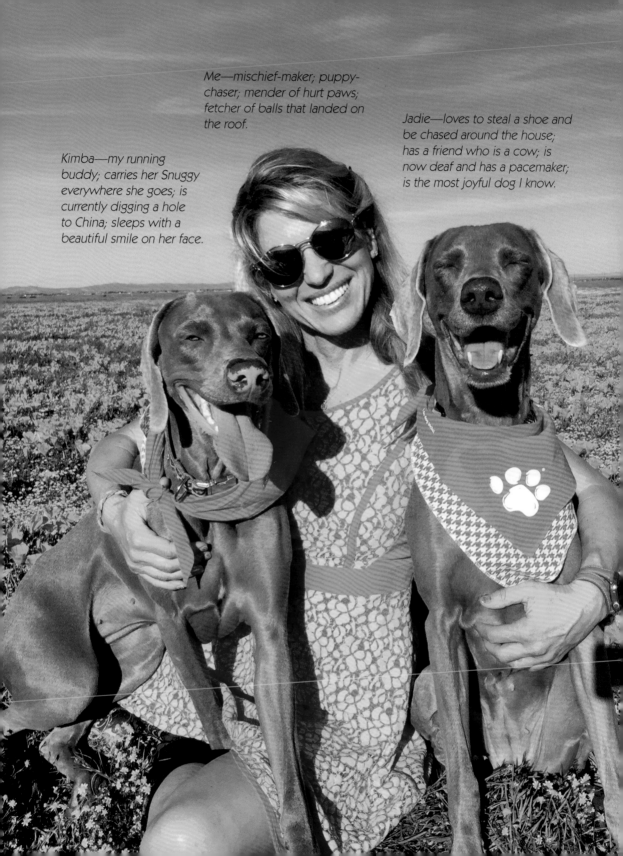

Me—mischief-maker; puppy-chaser; mender of hurt paws; fetcher of balls that landed on the roof.

Kimba—my running buddy; carries her Snuggy everywhere she goes; is currently digging a hole to China; sleeps with a beautiful smile on her face.

Jadie—loves to steal a shoe and be chased around the house; has a friend who is a cow; is now deaf and has a pacemaker; is the most joyful dog I know.

Teaching Skills and Sparking Enthusiasm!

One of the great joys in life is having the opportunity to spark a light in someone and to experience the excitement that comes with their new comprehension. We may have been lucky enough to experience this when coaching a sports team, showing a child how to ride a bike, or teaching a student to multiply fractions. That moment when they "get it," when the spark of comprehension ignites, is exciting, invigorating, and yes—*joyful.* It is a moment of connecting with another being on this earth, of achieving a goal. It's a laugh-out-loud, high-five, hip-hip-hooray moment! It's a moment you may retell later that evening with a smile on your face. It's a little thing; a tiny flower in a vast meadow. But flowers bloom one at a time, and if we are very lucky, and we give thoughtful attention to the cultivation of those little flowers, we will have a vibrant, effervescent field beneath our feet.

"Our brightest blazes are commonly kindled by unexpected sparks." —Samuel Johnson

Overcoming Our Roadblocks

You may have tried dog training in the past, and it may not have turned out as well as you'd hoped. Why was that? Was it too hard? Were the instructions unclear, wordy, or boring? Did you get frustrated? Were you not good at it and decided to quit rather than be less than perfect? Did it use methods that weren't fun for you and your dog? Good news—*The Joy of Dog Training* will be a different experience. You and your dog will have fun learning correct methods and be successful at achieving your goals.

It's Not Easy Being a Dog

Your life is full; you have your work, your friends, your hobbies. Your dog has only you. You are their source of companionship, of love, protection, and learning. Your dog has feelings just like you do. Your dog wants happiness; is hungry, bored, or hurting; has desires and hopes just like you do. Try looking at the world through their eyes—it's not easy being a dog. Through this book we will enrich our dog's life, and we will do it in a way that is loving, compassionate, encouraging, and forgiving. We will bring joy to our dog and, thereby, to ourselves as well.

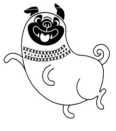

"It is amazing how much love and laughter they bring into our lives and even how much closer we become with each other because of them." —Josh Grogan

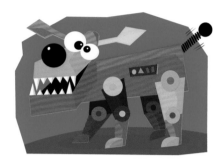

Dog Training Is an Art and a Science

When we become frustrated with training our dog, it's not because our dog is being bad or being stubborn. We get frustrated because we don't know what we're doing. We're frustrated because we've tried every technique we can think of, and none of them have worked. But we can choose a different way. *The Joy of Dog Training* empowers you with a clear plan of action and the skills to implement it, making you feel confident and secure in your strategy.

The Joy of Dog Training puts joy and positive reinforcement at the forefront; every method we use and tactic we employ will start with the premise of adding joy to our lives and to the lives of our dogs. We will use all positive methods to teach our dogs in a collaborative, fear-free environment that inspires our dog's willingness to learn. These methods yield fast results and a true, loving partnership.

While imparting sound, scientific training strategies, this book simultaneously employs colorful graphics, joyful photos, and encouraging quotes. It will keep you in a positive mindset, call your attention to good things and small gains in life, and remind you that regardless of the outcome, the joy is in the journey.

Through this book you will learn 30 animal training principles in bite-sized chunks—concepts such as **Reward Markers**, **Prompts**, **Shaping**, **Impulse Control**, and **Positive Redirection**. Each training principle is paired with easy-to-follow, step-by-step photo instructions demonstrating how to teach a trick using that principle, allowing you to practice and reinforce what you just learned.

Don't be fooled by the simple style of this book . . . it features academically sound, effective dog training principles used by elite trainers—presented with a joyful attitude!

ME:

MY DOG(S):

Long Live Joy!

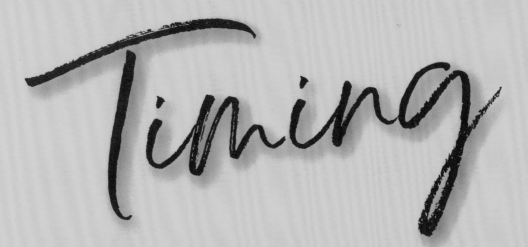

Timing

THE BASIS OF ANIMAL TRAINING

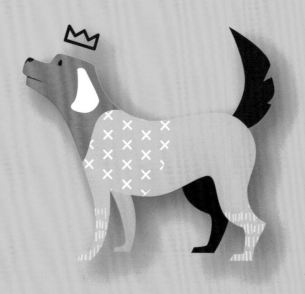

Dogs are intuitive and can form strong relationships with us, which allows us to be less than precise with our training methods. However, understanding the science behind animal training will make training faster, less frustrating, and more joyful for the both of you.

This chapter focuses on the core concepts of animal training. You will learn how to effectively communicate a goal behavior to your dog by rewarding them with correct **timing** and **positioning**; by using **reward markers** and **prompting**; and by evaluating and adjusting the criteria for success.

After learning each new lesson, you will have an opportunity to practice your new skill and reinforce the lesson by using the skill to teach your dog a trick.

Are you ready to get started?

Choose joy. Choose happy. Choose to shine!

Get Prepared with Training Tools

A few pieces of proper training gear will make your sessions go more smoothly.

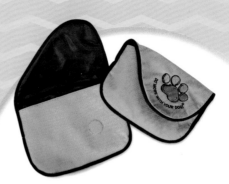

TREAT BAG

A waist-clip treat bag gives you quick access to treats without digging in your pockets.

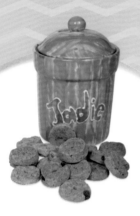

TREATS

Use tiny, soft treats that your dog can swallow quickly, such as hot dogs, meatballs, or chicken.

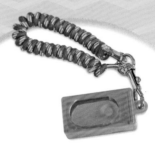

CLICKER

A dog training clicker makes a distinct sound that is an indicator of a correct behavior.

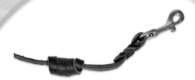

SHORT TAB LEAD

A simple grab tab hangs from your dog's collar. It does not get tangled, as a leash might, yet still gives you control when you need it.

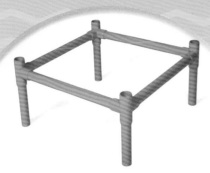

MAGIC SQUARE

A shallow pen used to confine a dog's front feet in a stay or as a destination to send the dog to.

TOY MOTIVATOR

Although we mostly train with treats, if your dog has a favorite ball or tug toy this can be an additional reward.

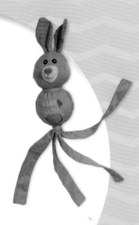

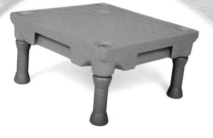

PEDESTAL

A raised platform is used as a home base to keep your dog focused and under control.

A GOOD ATTITUDE!

The most important training tool of all is your praise and encouragement!

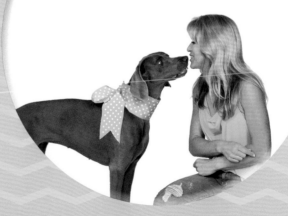

Reward at the Correct Time

The key to teaching any
behavior is to reward
success the instant your dog
performs correctly.
Be quick!

With humans, we can explain the connection between a behavior and its consequence, even if they are separated in time. For example, we can reward a child with dessert for having cleaned her room earlier. With dogs, we can't explain the connection between the behavior and the consequence. This is why the consequence has to be *immediate* in order for the dog to link it to the behavior.

During the learning process, your dog may be squirming and trying a variety of different things. You need to let them know immediately whether each thing they try is a success (treat) or nonsuccess (no treat). Your job is to make sure they understand exactly what it was that they did to earn that treat, and the key to helping them understand the goal behavior is to **give the treat at the exact moment that they perform correctly**.

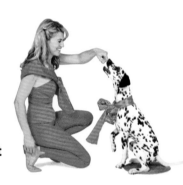

If you are teaching your dog to sit, for example, you'll want to pop that treat in their mouth at the exact moment when their rear drops to the floor.

"Never trust people who don't have something in their lives that they love beyond all reason."
—*Fredrik Backman*

Let's practice this lesson by teaching:

Touch My Hand

Let's teach our dog to nose-touch our hand. We will help them understand the goal behavior by **rewarding them at the correct time**—giving them the treat the instant that they nose-touch our hand. Through the use of precise timing, your dog will make the association between the action and the reward and will know exactly what they are being rewarded for. Smiles and excited praise will speed up learning even more!

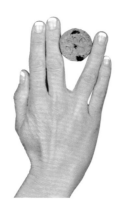

1 **WEDGE A TREAT BETWEEN YOUR FINGERS**

Choose a yummy, smelly treat that will entice your dog to investigate.

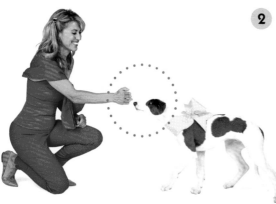

2 **HOLD OUT YOUR HAND**

Say, "Touch!" and hold your palm toward your dog, at nose height. Don't push your hand at your dog, but rather wait for your dog to come to your hand.

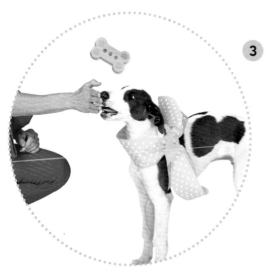

3 **RELEASE THE TREAT**

The instant your dog touches your hand, release the treat. See how fast they learn this trick!

Reward in the Correct Position

When teaching a new behavior, give the reward while your dog is in the correct position.

When a dog recieves a reward, they associate their current body position with earning the treat. If you are teaching your dog to sit, give them the treat while they are are in the **correct position**— sitting.

Formulate a clear image in your head of what your dog looks like in the correct position. Then put that image into words. That way you will be quick to react when you see your dog in that correct position. When teaching Paws Up, you might think, "Both paws are on the platform." Shake Hands might be "Their paw rests in my hand." On the next page we will teach Sit. How would you describe the correct body position for Sit?

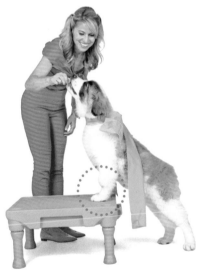

PAWS UP

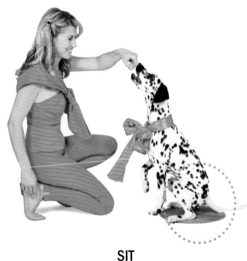

SIT

Let's practice this lesson by teaching:

Sit

Some dogs move very quickly. When learning a sit, they may drop their rear to the floor for only a second before standing up again. We want, as much as possible, for your dog to have the experience of being **rewarded while in the correct position**. We want them to eat the treat while their rear is still touching the floor. In order to make this happen, you will have to carefully control the placement of your hand as they are eating. You can even let them nibble the treat from your hand for a few seconds while they remain sitting.

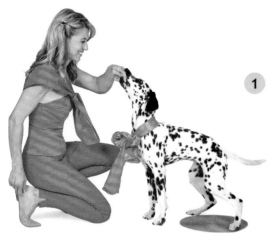

1 HOLD A TREAT ABOVE THEIR HEAD

Hold a treat above your dog's head, and let them sniff and nibble at it.

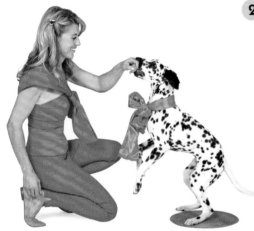

2 MOVE THE TREAT BACK

Slowly move the treat backward toward their tail, which should cause their rear to drop. If they jump or back up, it may help to have a wall behind them. It may take a few minutes of squirming until your dog sits.

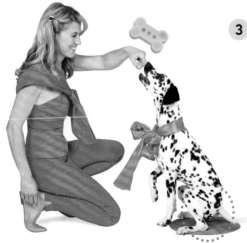

3 REWARD IN THE CORRECT POSITION

When your dog's rear hits the floor, release the treat. It may help to have several treats in your hand and let your dog nibble them so long as they maintain sitting. Introduce the verbal cue by saying, "Good sit."

Reward Markers & Clickers

Use a reward marker to inform your dog of the exact moment they achieved the goal behavior and earned a treat.

We know that in the learning stage it is important to reward our dog at the exact moment they perform correctly. The timing of the treat marks the exact moment the dog performs the goal behavior. This **mark** helps the dog understand which behavior they need to repeat.

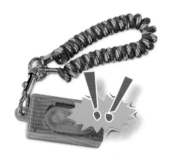

But it is sometimes logistically difficult to get a treat in our dog's mouth at the exact right moment. If your dog is learning to jump through a hoop, for example, you wouldn't be able to toss a treat in their mouth at the exact moment they intersect the hoop. We need another way to **mark** that instant of success. So we mark it with a sound. We use a specific sound (such as the *click-click* of a dog training clicker) to identify the instant the dog performed the goal behavior and earned a reward. We call this specific sound a **reward marker**, because it marks the instant the dog earned a reward.

Every reward marker (click) is quickly followed by a reward (treat).

There's always something to celebrate!

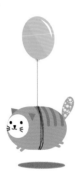

EVERY FORM OF ANIMAL TRAINING RELIES ON REWARD MARKERS

Whether they realize it or not, every successful animal trainer is using reward markers. The reward marker may be a deliberate sound or word such as *click-click* or "Good!" or a less conscious use of praise.

Reward markers are used in all forms of animal training. Marine mammal trainers use a whistle as a reward marker; horse trainers use a tongue pop; and other trainers may use a finger snap or a special word. Many dog trainers use a handheld **clicker**, a thumb-size box with a metal tongue that makes a *click-click* sound when pressed. A wrist strap or lanyard will keep it easily accessible.

One of the advantages of the clicker sound, which has traditionally been used in zoos in the training of exotic animals and in training animal actors for movies and TV, is its ability to be standardized across all trainers working with an animal.

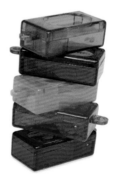

> **MY REWARD MARKER WORD:**

CAN I USE A SPECIAL WORD INSTEAD OF A CLICKER?

You absolutely can, and many trainers do. Common reward makers words are "Good!" and "Yes," but you can choose whatever word makes you happy. Although it is logistically easier to use a unique word as a reward marker rather than a handheld clicker, a clicker does have advatages of precision timing, consistent sound, and absence of emotion.

Precision Timing: The clicker sound is very short, crisp, and distinct and can mark a precise instant. If you chose a verbal reward marker, make it short and crisp. Novice trainers commonly have a quicker reaction time with a clicker than with their special word.

Consistent Sound: Novice trainers may vocalize their reward marker word differently depending upon their mood. Clickers always sound exactly the same.

Absence of Emotion: Dogs are sensitive to our moods and can be upset by frustration in our voice. A clicker separates the marker from any frustration or other emotion you may be feeling. It allows the dog to focus on what *they* are doing rather than worrying about how your mood is changing. Don't underestimate the importance of this point— it's one of the main advantages of the clicker.

Let's practice this lesson by teaching:

Touch a Target Disc

In lesson 1 we taught our dog to nose-touch our hand. Now we will build on that skill to teach our dog to nose-touch a disc. In lesson 1 we used a treat to mark the instant our dog performed correctly. In this lesson we will **click a clicker** to mark the instant our dog performs correctly. Remember that the click is a signal that your dog just earned a treat. Follow every click with a treat.

If your dog is "sound shy" and startled by the clicker, use your reward marker word instead.

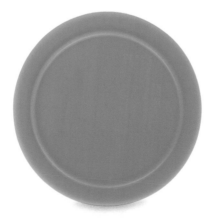

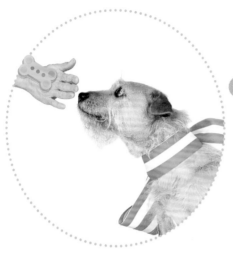

1 REVIEW "TOUCH MY HAND"

Do a few iterations of **Touch My Hand** (page 18), rewarding your dog with the treat from between your fingers.

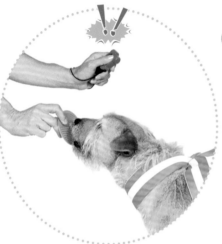

2 HOLD OUT THE DISC AND CLICK

Rub some treats on the disc to get your dog's interest. Hold the disc in one hand and your clicker and a treat in the other. Say, "Touch!" The instant they touch the disc, click your clicker.

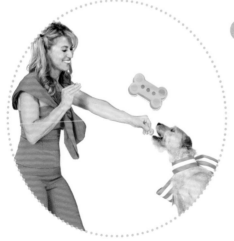

3 FOLLOW EACH CLICK WITH A TREAT

Follow each click with a treat in order to maintain the efficacy of this tool. You now have a way to mark correct behavior!

Progression

Once your dog is achieving success, increase the criteria and ask for a more advanced version of the behavior.

The purpose of a treat is to reward a good effort. In kindergarten, a child gets a gold star for printing their name. In first grade, they only get a gold star if they print it neatly, and in second grade, cursive is required for that same reward. What earned your dog a treat in the past may no longer be enough to earn that treat today. We call this **progression**.

On the next page you will teach your dog to step inside a box. When first teaching them this trick, you may reward them for placing just one paw in the box. As they get the hang of this, you will progress to requiring more, withholding the treat until they place both paws in the box.

Every time your dog is achieving a step with about 75 percent success, require a higher skill to earn the treat.

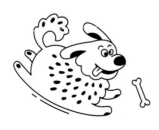

The goal of each training session is to get results a little better than the last time.

Let's practice this lesson by teaching:

Paws in a Box

This is a confidence-building exercise for your dog as you coax them to place their paws in a Magic Square (page 14) or in a box. In the beginning, reward your dog for placing just one paw in the box. Over time, **progress** and ask more of them.

You may use your clicker to mark the correct behavior, or you may simply deliver the treat at the moment your dog achieves your criteria.

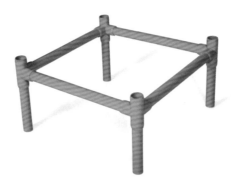

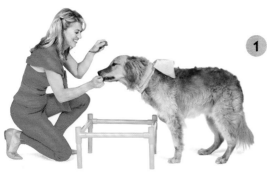

1 LURE YOUR DOG FORWARD

Gently coax your dog forward by allowing them to lick a tasty treat from your hand and then moving the treat just out of their reach.

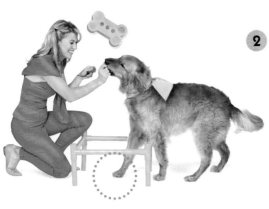

2 ONE FOOT IN THE BOX

Your dog may put one paw in the box and quickly remove it. Reward them while they are in the **correct position**.

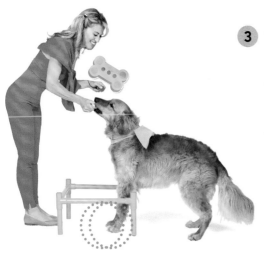

3 TWO FEET IN THE BOX

Once your dog seems to understand the goal behavior, it's time to **progress**. Coax them forward and withold the treat until they put *both* feet in the box. Nice!

Regression

When your dog is struggling, take a step back; temporarily lower the criteria for success.

The key to keeping your dog motivated is to keep them challenged and achieving regular successes. This requires a constant shift between **progressing** by asking for a more difficult behavior and **regressing** by asking for an easier behavior.

Try not to let your dog be wrong more than two or three times in a row or they could become discouraged and not wish to perform. If your dog is struggling, temporarily lower the criteria for success. Go back to an easier step where they can be successful for a while.

The process of learning a behavior is not linear. Your dog will go through numerous spurts of progression and regression. Don't be reluctant to go back a step—it's usually only needed for a short while and will give your dog confidence to move forward.

No matter what the issue, never push ahead in the training process if you reach a point where your dog is not confident. Instead, back up a few steps to where your dog showed the greatest degree of confidence and build their skills from there.

Strive for progress, not perfection.

Let's practice this lesson by teaching:

Send to a Mark

Movie dogs are taught to go to a mark—to step on a disc on the floor. This same skill is used to send a dog to their spot (their bed or home base) or to teach a dog a trick such as stepping on a tap light to turn it on.

Your dog has already learned to put their paws in a box (page 32). We will now build on that skill to teach them to step on a mark. Through this process your dog will go through periods of progression as well as **regression**. If they are struggling, regress back to an easier step.

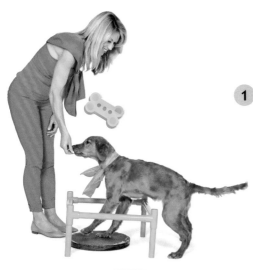

1 BUILD ON PAWS IN A BOX

Place a mark (preferably one with a little height) inside your box or Magic Square. Use a treat to lure in your dog. Reward them for stepping on the mark.

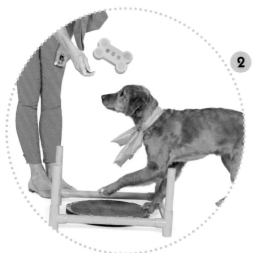

2 LOWER THE PROFILE OF THE BOX

Turn your Magic Square upside down or reduce the profile of your box. Again, lure your dog to step on the mark and reward them while they are in the **correct position**: stepping on the mark.

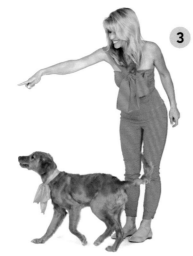

3 REMOVE THE BOX

Remove the box or Magic Square and send your dog to the mark with a wave of your arm. If they have trouble and are unsuccessul two or three times in a row, **regress** back to a previous step.

Is Your Dog Right-Pawed or Left-Pawed?

Like humans, most dogs have a paw preference; they are either right-pawed or left-pawed. To find your dog's paw preference, take note of which paw they favor in daily activities. When they walk down stairs, with which paw do they lead? Which paw do they use to scratch at the door or your leg?

Some dogs show no significant paw preference. These dogs have significantly more noise phobias, reacting strongly to thunderstorms and fireworks. A similar finding in humans has shown a correlation between people with weaker hand preferences and extreme anxiety.

STEP IN A BOX
When stepping into or onto something, with which foot does your dog lead?

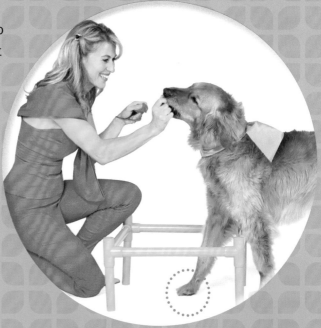

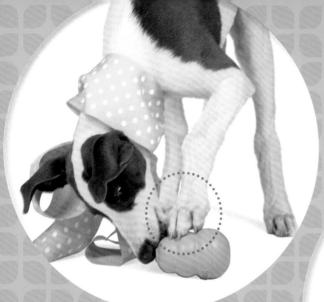

PEANUT-BUTTER TOY

Which paw does your dog use to hold down a bone or toy filled with peanut butter?

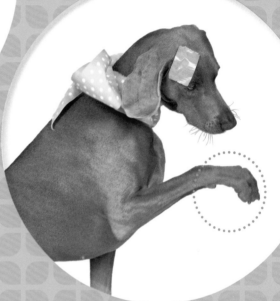

TAPE

Which paw does your dog use to swipe off a piece of tape stuck to their head?

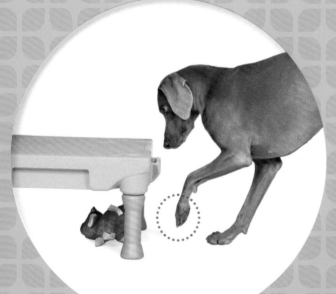

TOY UNDER SOFA

When your dog's toy gets pushed under the sofa, which paw do they use to pull it out?

Teach Verbal Cues

Teach your dog to respond to a verbal cue word through the repetition of cue, pause, prompt, reward.

So far you've been using a treat to lure your dog into a sit. We will now teach your dog to sit in response to just your verbal cue. When you say "Sit," your dog will sit.

A **cue** is the word we use to ask for the behavior (such as the word "Sit"). A **prompt** is a more invasive hint to the dog (such using a treat to lure them into a sit or pressing down on their rear).

When we teach a new verbal cue to a dog, we do it in the sequence of **cue**, **pause**, **prompt**, **reward**. First we say "Sit" (**cue**), then we **pause** to give the dog a chance to do the behavior, and if they don't, we give a more helpful **prompt** (such as luring their head or pressing down on their rear). As soon as the dog sits, they get a **reward**.

The pause is very important. The dog wants the treat as quickly as possible, so they will try to anticipate the goal behavior. Eventually the dog will start to perform the behavior during the pause. Success!

1 CUE
Say the cue

2 PAUSE
Pause to
let it sink in

3 PROMPT
Give a hint

4 REWARD
Reward with
a treat

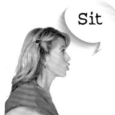
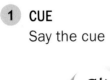
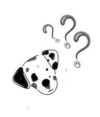
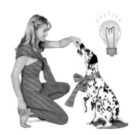

Let's practice this lesson by teaching:

Introduce a Verbal Cue

In lesson 5, your dog learned to go to a mark. We will now progress the criteria on that behavior and teach your dog to go to a mark while responding to just a **verbal cue**.

We will first give the verbal **cue**, **pause**, **prompt** your dog (by moving toward the mark and pointing at it), and then **reward**. Over time, your dog will learn to run to the mark as soon as they hear your verbal cue.

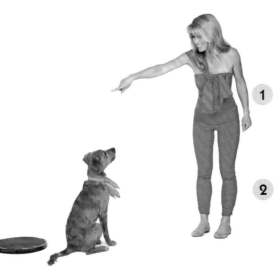

1 **CUE**

Say, "Target." Your dog won't know what this means yet.

2 **PAUSE**

Let it sink in for a second.

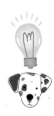

3 **PROMPT**

Give helpful **prompts** to your dog to get them to step on the mark.

4 **REWARD**

Give your dog a treat while they are in the **correct position**; standing on the mark. You can even repeat "Good target" to further emphasize this new cue word.

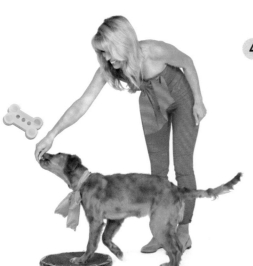

Visual Guide to Hand Signals

Hand signals can cue behaviors. Most dogs respond to hand signals even more readily than verbal cues.

Dogs can perform a behavior in response to a **verbal cue** or a **hand signal cue**. Hand signals are standardized in industries such as animal acting so that any trainer can work a dog. They are not arbitrary; they are usually born out of the initial luring pattern used when first training the dog. The raising of the hand as a signal to sit evolves from your initial upward luring when teaching the behavior. A downward hand motion is used to signal "down" and parallels your initial luring of your dog near the floor (see page 62). And a flick of your wrist is a diminished version of the large circle you will draw when teaching your dog to spin (see page 52).

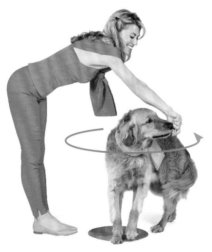
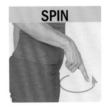

SPIN

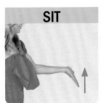

SIT

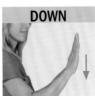

DOWN

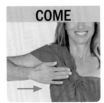

COME

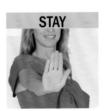

STAY

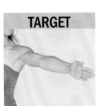

TARGET

Technique

THE SIX TOOLS IN OUR TOOLBOX

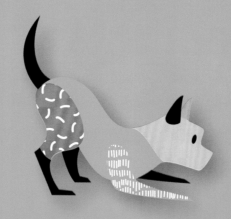

We've learned the importance of rewarding our dog with **correct timing** and **correct positioning**. We've gotten our dog to perform a behavior and then rewarded it. But the real challenge is often in figuring out *how* to get our dog to do the behavior in the first place!

As dog trainers, we have at our disposal **six techniques** for eliciting a behavior. In this chapter, we will explore each of those techniques by training a trick using that method.

All methods of getting the behavior are not equal, and none is right for every trainer, every dog, and every situation. Pay attention to which techniques feel best for you and produce the best results with your dog. These are the tools we have in our toolkit, but sometimes the best solution uses a combination of techniques.

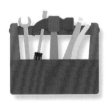

It is neccessary to have good tools, but it is also neccessary to use the tools in the right way.

The Six Ways to Elicit a Behavior

In order to teach a dog a behavior, we have to reward them. And in order to reward them, we have to get them to do the behavior. So how do we get them to do the behavior for the first time?

When teaching sit we may **lure** our dog into position with a treat, or we may **press down** on their rear. But not all tricks have solutions that obvious. How would we, for example, teach a dog to hold an object in their mouth? Or to speak on cue? How about to put their toy in a toy box or to press a button with their paw? Search-and-rescue dogs may have to track a person's scent trail, and animal actors might be asked to yawn on cue. If these behaviors have you stumped, take comfort—the solution to every behavior training challenge lies in your six tools. Learn how to use these tools and you'll be able to teach any behavior.

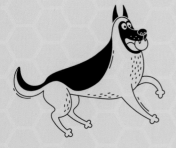

With imagination, simple tools can create remarkable results.

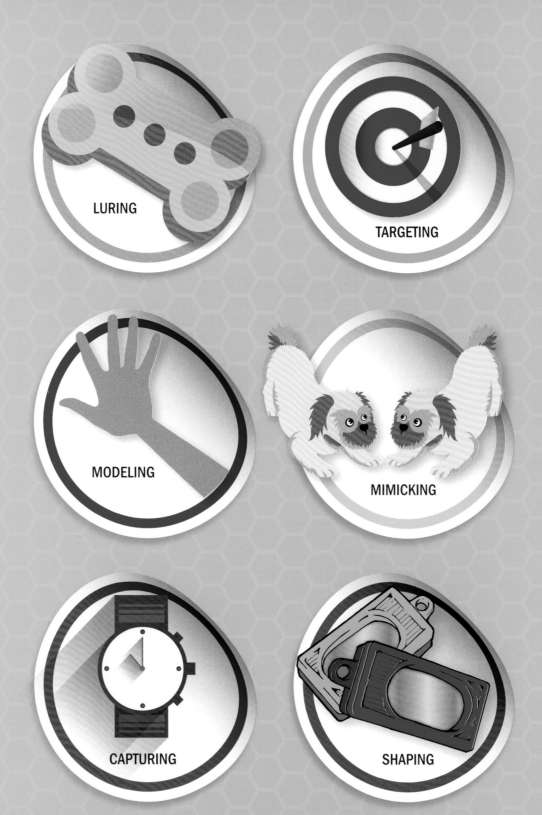

LURING

TARGETING

MODELING

MIMICKING

CAPTURING

SHAPING

Luring

Luring is the technique of encouraging a dog to follow a treat to get them in the correct position.

Luring is the most common technique used to teach behaviors; we use a treat to guide the dog's nose, and the rest of their body will follow. We've already used luring to teach several tricks. In **Touch My Hand** we held a treat between our fingers to lure the dog to touch our palm. When teaching **Sit** we moved a treat over the dog's head, causing their nose to point up and their rear to drop. We pulled the treat forward to lead them in **Paws in a Box** and **Send to a Mark**.

Luring is fast, flexible, and precise. It's easy to learn for both the trainer and the dog. Although many dog tricks are taught by luring, not every trick can be taught by this technique. Luring just guides the head, and hopefully the body will follow. You can't teach a dog to bark, to fetch, or to catch a flying disc with luring.

Clickers and reward marker words are superfluous with luring. The treat acts as the **marker** and is given at the instant the behavior happens. A clicker imparts no additional information. Let's try this technique to teach a trick!

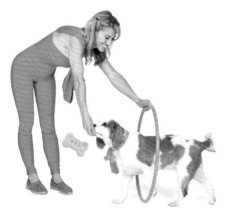

GO THROUGH A HOOP

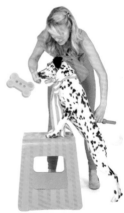

PAWS UP

Let's practice this lesson by teaching:

Spin Circles

We will use the **luring** technique to teach our dog to spin circles. We use a treat to guide their head in a large circle and hopefully their body will follow! Move your hand slowly when luring so as not to lose your dog's nose.

We eventually want to **fade the lure** and be able to get the behavior without a treat in our hand. We do this by doing several iterations with a treat in our hand, followed by one try using just our pointed finger as a lure. As usual, give a reward at the end of the circle.

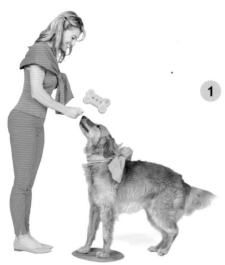

1 SHOW THE LURE TO YOUR DOG

Hold several small treats at your dog's nose height. Say the **verbal cue**, "Spin."

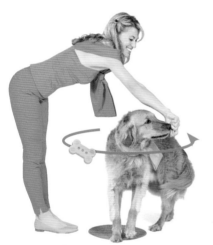

2 MOVE IT IN A BIG CIRCLE

Slowly move the **lure** in a big circle. If your dog loses interest, let them have some of the treats along the way.

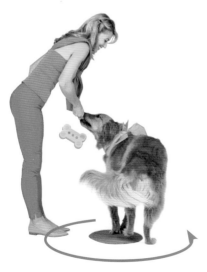

3 AT THE END, RELEASE A TREAT

The release of the treat lets your dog know that they achieved the goal behavior.

Let's practice this lesson by teaching:

Paws Up

Let's try another trick using the **luring** technique: teaching our dog to put their front paws up on an object.

The **lure** is our tool. We want our tool to be a strong one—an enticement to our dog—so we will want to use extra-yummy dog treats or even people food such as ham, chicken, steak, popcorn, pizza crusts, or cheese.

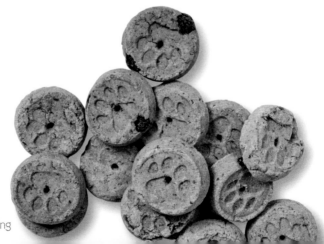

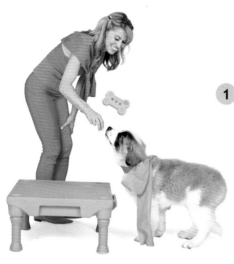

1 PRESENT THE LURE

Hold several treats slightly above a sturdy piece of furniture and cue your dog, "Paws up." Pat the item to coax your dog's front feet onto it.

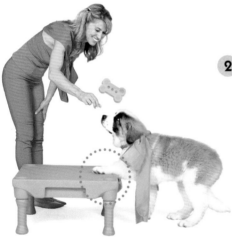

2 MOVE THE LURE JUST OUT OF REACH

As your dog reaches for the **lure**, let them have a small taste of the treat and then move it just out of their reach. Give them verbal encouragement to follow it.

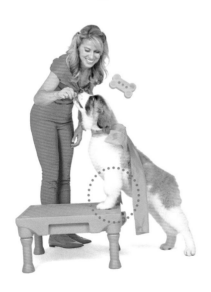

3 SUCCESS!

When both paws are on the box, let them have the reward. Remember to reward while the dog remains in the **correct position**.

Targeting

A target stick is an extension of a lure. The dog learns to nose-touch the end of the stick, and we use this to guide them into position.

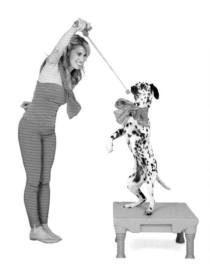

We've practiced using a treat to **lure** our dog into position. A **target stick** is another kind of luring device. This stick has a ball or cup at the end, which we teach the dog to nose-touch. By moving the end of the stick, we guide our dog to follow it.

A target stick allows us to have a longer reach, thus making it logistically easier to guide a small dog to spin a circle or a large dog to lie down. This gives us more options with our dog, and, once taught, gives us a useful tool in our toolbox.

Target sticks are also a safe way to lure a dog who likes to nip at your fingers.

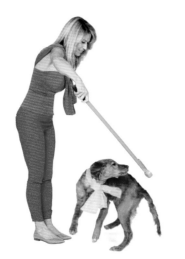

SPIN CIRCLES

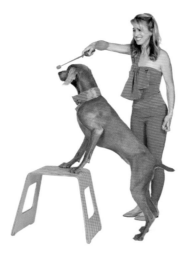

PAWS UP

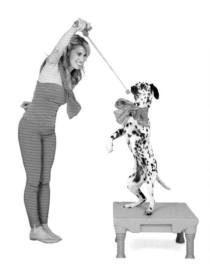

STAND TALL

Let's practice this lesson by teaching:

Touch a Target Stick

Anything we can teach with luring we can also teach with **targeting**. A target stick is merely an extension of your arm. A telescoping back scratcher offers a convenient, portable option for making a target stick. Affix a small ball to the end of the stick for the touch object.

In this lesson we will teach your dog to target by affixing a measuring cup to the end of a stick. The cup has the advantage of being able to hold a treat, which we will use as both the lure and the reward. Use a wet treat, such as a hot dog slice, in the cup (hard kibble tends to bounce out of the cup at inconvenient times).

Because we are not giving the treat at the exact moment the dog touches the target stick, we will click our **clicker** at that moment and follow up with a treat.

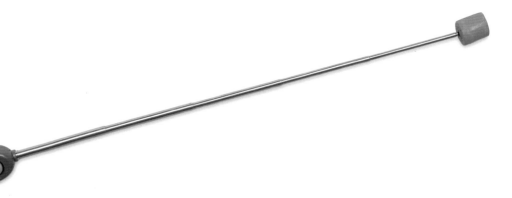

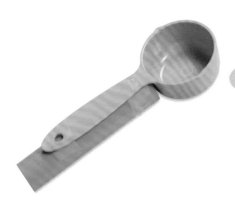

1 MAKE A TARGET STICK

Attach a measuring cup to a pole.

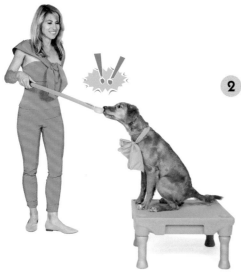

2 CLICK THE TOUCH

Put a treat in the cup and show it to your dog. Tell them, "Touch!" Let them come to the cup rather than pushing the cup toward them. When they touch the cup, click your **clicker**.

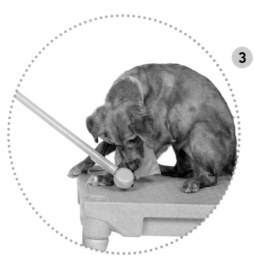

3 DISPENSE THE TREAT

Remember, **every click is immediately followed by a treat**. Empty the cup to let your dog have the treat.

Build on Known Behaviors

Once your dog has a foundation of core behaviors, you can build on those skills to more easily teach new tricks. Here are some ways to build on the skills your dog has learned so far.

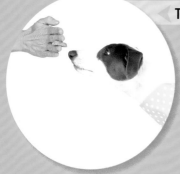

TOUCH MY HAND

Once your dog knows Touch My Hand, hold out your hand and call, "Come!"

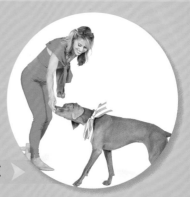

COME

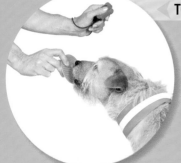

TOUCH A DISC

Once your dog knows Touch a Target Disc, tape the disc onto a ball.

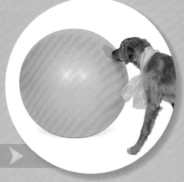

PUSH A BALL

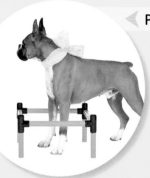

PAWS IN A BOX

With your dog's paws in the box, use a treat to lure their head down into a bow.

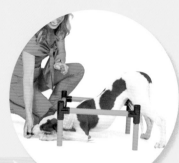

TAKE A BOW

SEND TO A MARK

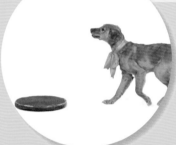

It's an easy transition from sending to a mark to sending to a home base.

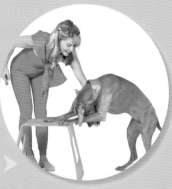

GO TO YOUR HOME BASE

PAWS UP

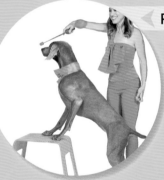

With your dog's paws up, use a treat to lure their head to their chest.

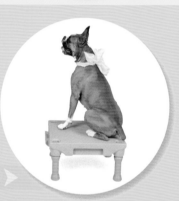

SAY YOUR PRAYERS

TARGET STICK

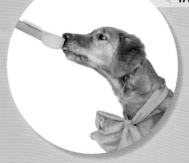

Lower the target stick between your dog's front paws to get them to lie down.

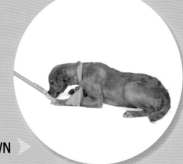

DOWN

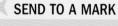

Modeling

Modeling is the technique of physically guiding or manipulating a dog into position.

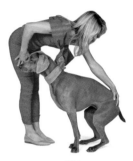

Probably the most obvious method of eliciting a behavior is through **modeling**. In modeling, we use our hand or a prop to either touch the dog or create a barrier that compels the desired behavior.

SIT

Examples of modeling would be pushing down on a dog's rear to compel a sit, pushing on their shoulder to compel them to lie down, pulling on their leash to teach them to walk at heel, and putting our palm in front of their nose to get them to stay. We generally only model the core part of a dog's body and do so to produce large behaviors such as sit, down, heel, and stay.

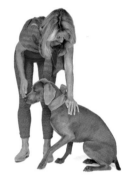

DOWN

It is tempting to manipulate your dog's body physically because it feels like we can get the behavior faster. **Modeling, however, can actually delay the learning process**. By manipulating your dog, you are encouraging them to relinquish initiative and to be led. They are not required to engage their brain and figure out how to position their body by themselves.

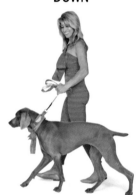

HEEL

When modeling, use the minimum amount of pressure needed at every stage of learning. You want to use your touch as a hint, or reminder, and let your dog come up with the behavior on their own.

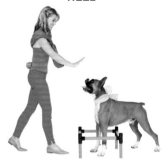

STAY

Let's practice this lesson by teaching:

Stay in a Square

One of the problems we may encounter when teaching our dog to stay is that they creep forward, taking subtle baby steps. With the **modeling** technique, we will use a Magic Square to contain their feet and help them understand they need to stay put. The square acts as a **boundary**, compelling their behavior.

Use firm body language to help hold your dog's stay. Stand up straight and make steady eye contact with your dog. Your hand signals should be rigid and meaningful.

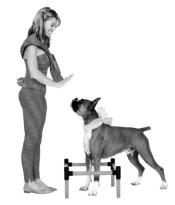
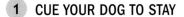

1 CUE YOUR DOG TO STAY

Lure your dog to put their front paws in the square. Hold a treat behind your back. Say, "Stay" and give the signal with your other hand.

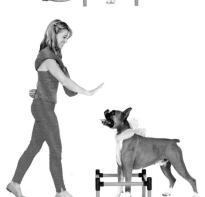
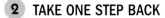

2 TAKE ONE STEP BACK

Keep your hand firmly in the stay signal and take one step back.

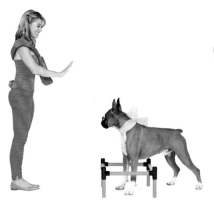

3 WAIT A SECOND

Hold your dog with eye contact and firm body posture. Keep your hand signal up to steady them.

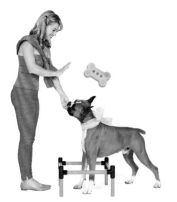

4 TAKE ONE STEP FORWARD

Keep your hand signal up. Do not draw out the treat hand from behind your back until a second after you have returned to your dog. Reward while they are in the **correct position**.

Mimicking

Mimicry is the tendency of a dog to copy the behavior of a trainer or another dog.

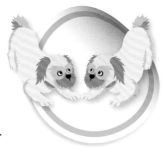

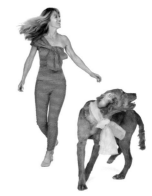

Dogs will learn from other dogs.
If you pair an untrained dog
with a dog who has a terrific recall, the untrained
dog will learn to follow the model of the trained dog.
It is common for novice herding dogs, hunting dogs,
and sled dogs to be paired with experienced dogs
who show them the ropes. The tendency to **mimic** is
particularly strong in half-grown puppies.

SPIN CIRCLES

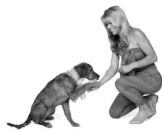

Some breeds are easier to train using mimicry than
others (herding breeds take to it easily), and it varies
between individual dogs. Mimicry works best with
natural behaviors, such as howling together, barking,
walking together, fetching, or engaging in play
behavior.

SHAKE HANDS

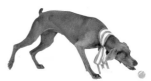

Depending on the dog, you can sometimes get them
to mimic other behaviors, such as spinning circles,
shaking your hand, crawling, or tugging.

FETCH

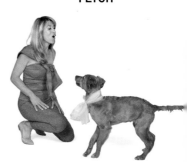

BARK

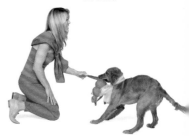

TUG

Let's practice this lesson by teaching:

Jump over a Bar

Jumping is a fun behavior, and it's even more fun when you do it together! We'll use the technique of **mimicry** to get our dog to jump over a bar.

Mimicry works best when your dog is enticed into the behavior with enthusiasm and play behavior. Make it a game, a competition; race your dog as you both hop over various obstacles. Encourage your dog with excited praise. Be joyful!

We can judge a person's character by how they treat their canine companion.

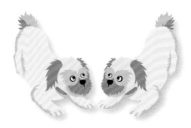

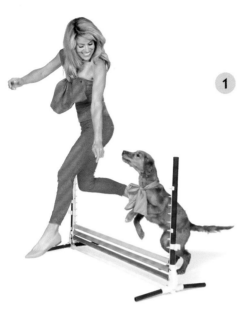

1 JUMP OVER A LOW BAR

Start with a low bar or even no bar at all. Get your dog excited and pat your leg to keep them near you as you hop over the bar. Did they **mimic**?

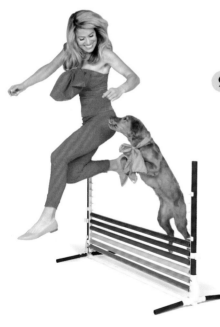

2 RAISE IT UP

Raise the height of the bar and leap over it. When it gets too high for you to safely jump, run instead to the side of it and wave your arm over the jump. Have fun!

Capturing

Capturing is the technique of waiting for the dog to do the behavior unprovoked and then rewarding that behavior.

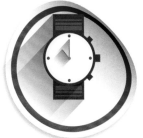

With **capturing**, we wait for our dog to do the goal behavior on their own, and then we give them a treat. With enough repetition, the dog will eventually learn to do the behavior on cue.

You can use the capturing technique to teach your dog to **bow**. Watch and wait for them to do this behavior naturally, such as when they wake from a nap and stretch. At that second, click your clicker or say your reward maker word, then give them a treat. Over time, they'll figure out that every time they bow, you give them a treat. Once they are **offering this behavior**, you can start to associate a verbal cue with it: "Bow."

Capturing is limited to naturally occurring behaviors; you probably won't capture your dog riding a skateboard or putting a basketball in a net. Capturing is also limited to behaviors that occur with enough frequency that the dog can figure out a pattern. For example, does your dog bark often enough that you can capture that behavior and assign it a **cue word**?

A little progress each day adds up to big results.

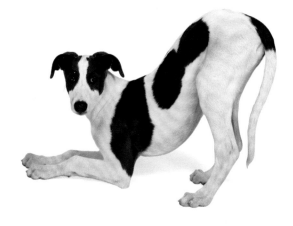

Let's practice this lesson by teaching:

Speak

We will teach our dog to bark on cue. Once they understand "Speak," we can also teach them "No speak" to get them to stop barking. We will teach this trick using the **capturing** technique, waiting until the dog does the behavior on their own and then rewarding it. But because we don't want to wait around all day, we are going to help the capturing process along by doing a little something to instigate that bark. What causes your dog to bark? A cat? Tapping on a window? Whatever it is that can cause a bark can be used to teach your dog to speak on cue. In this example, we'll use the doorbell to elicit a bark.

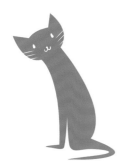

If it's worth doing, it's worth doing with enthusiasm!

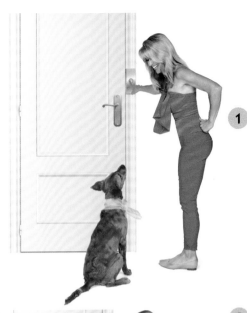

1 RING THE DOORBELL TO ELICIT A BARK

Stand outside your front door. Cue, "Speak!" and ring the doorbell. If your dog does not bark at first, try saying, "What was that?!"

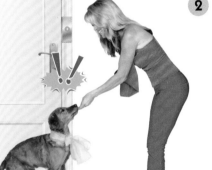

2 MARK AND REWARD

When you get a bark, mark the instant with your **clicker** or verbal **reward marker** word and follow up with a treat. Reinforce the cue word and speed up learning by saying, "Good speak."

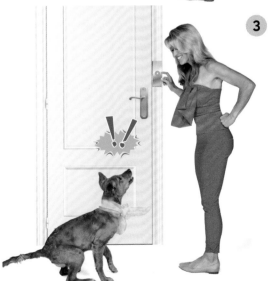

3 PRETEND TO THE RING THE DOORBELL

Say, "Speak!" and pretend to ring the doorbell. This may be enough to elicit the bark. Follow the bark with a click and a treat. If your dog doesn't bark, **regress** to step 1. Wean off of the doorbell quickly, as you don't want to inadvertently teach your dog to bark at it.

Shaping

Shaping is the technique of
building a new behavior by
rewarding baby steps that
come closer and closer to
the goal.

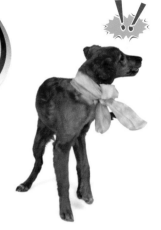

Shaping is essentially a game we play with our dog in which we have a goal behavior in mind that our dog tries to figure out. It's a little like the game in which one person wanders around while the other tells them if they are getting hotter or colder (closer to or farther away from the goal). Once a dog has experience with this game, it can allow them to quickly home in on a new behavior. It's a collaborative process and becomes a fun brain challenge for the both of you.

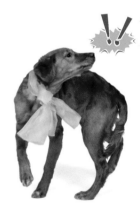

LOOK LEFT

With shaping, we don't do anything to elicit the behavior; we don't lure or physically manipulate the dog. We just stand back and wait to **capture** a baby step of the behavior and then reward it. We break the behavior into teeny-tiny, baby steps and start by rewarding the most basic component of the trick. **Clickers** are often used in the process of shaping to give instant feedback to the dog.

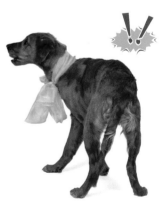

TAKE A STEP LEFT

Earlier, we used the **luring** technique to teach our dog to spin circles (page 52). We can also use the shaping technique to teach this trick. To do so, we would wait until our dog happened to barely move their head left, then we'd click and reward that. Eventually we'd **progress the criteria** and wait until they looked left and also took one step to the left, and we'd reward that. In baby steps, we'd eventually get them to walk all the way in a circle.

COMPLETE CIRCLE

Let's practice this lesson by teaching:

Pick Up a Toy

Some dogs readily pick up things in their mouths. Other dogs need to be taught this trick. We will use the technique of **shaping** to break down this trick into baby steps and reward each increment. Over time, we will get our dog to pick up a toy and hold it in their mouth.

You will go through a lot of treats in this first session; that's fine. Remember to be quick with your clicker and follow every click with a treat.

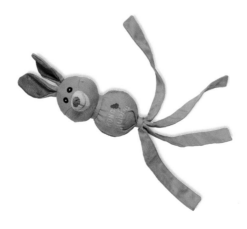

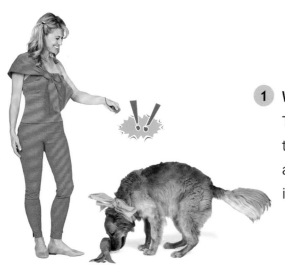

1 WAIT FOR YOUR DOG TO NOTICE THE TOY

The first step when using **shaping** is to click and reward your dog for taking any notice of the toy (even glancing at it). Do this a dozen times.

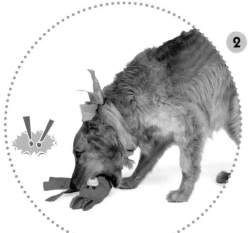

2 RAISE THE CRITERIA

Once your dog catches on, **progress** and require more from them to earn the treat. Withhold the click until they touch the toy, or nudge it, or mouth it. Follow each click with a treat.

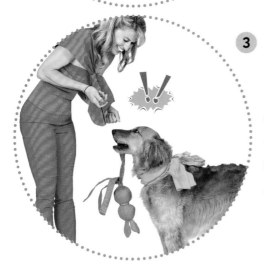

3 RAISE THE CRITERIA AGAIN

Every time your dog seems to get the hang of it, ask for a little more. You should be clicking and rewarding about every two to ten seconds. If your dog is struggling, **regress** to an easier step for a while.

Good Work!

Look at all you've learned! You're doing great. And your dog is awesome! Let's take a few minutes and bask in the memories of our good work and great times together.

Your dog has worked hard—recognize their accomplishments! Whether they've earned Best Barker or Most Improved Attitude, your dog deserves a special treat tonight.

MY DOG'S ACCOMPLISHMENT:

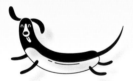

ASK YOUR DOG THESE QUESTIONS AND WRITE DOWN THEIR ANSWERS.

Do you like when we train together? Do you want to do more of it?

Who is your best friend?

Do you forgive me for all the mistakes I've made (and those I will make in the future)?

MY PROMISE TO MY DOG:

When I become frustrated during training, I will:

When I compare you to other dogs, I will remember:

I will think of your needs, even when:

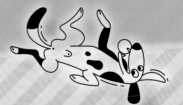

"*The most wasted of all days is one without laughter.*"

—Nicolas Chamfort

MEASURE YOUR DOG'S SUCCESS NOT ONLY BY THE TRICKS THEY HAVE LEARNED BUT ALSO BY IMPROVED ATTENTION AND WORK ETHIC.

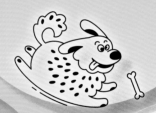

My dog enjoys training this trick:

Something new I learned about my dog:

I'm really proud of my dog for:

My dog's nickname is:

The main rewards my dog works for are:

What has your dog done lately to make you laugh and smile?

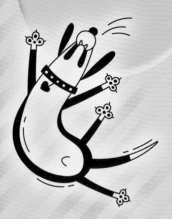

Motivation

PRINCIPLES OF POSITIVE REINFORCEMENT

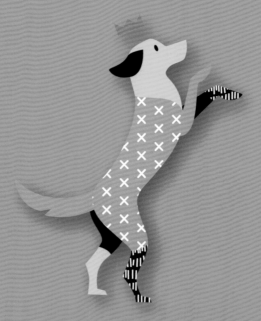

Out of all the dog training books on the shelf, why did you choose this one? Perhaps it's because you are dedicated to the idea of your dog as a family member and are committed to training with **compassion** and gentleness. Your aim is not to suppress behavior and teach subservience but rather to have a **joyful** relationship with a confident and happy dog who is motivated to do the right thing rather than fearful of making a mistake.

In this chapter you will learn how to get the quickest learning with the highest rate of retention through the use of **positive reinforcement** training. You will learn how to set up your dog for success to foster a trusting relationship. And you will identify **motivators** for your dog and learn how to use them as rewards to drive behavior.

Behavior becomes a habit, and as you and your dog learn to operate in a rewards-based relationship, you will find that every aspect of your life together begins to reflect this joyful disposition.

Nine-tenths of dog training is encouragement.

You Owe This to Your Dog

Our dogs play significant roles in our lives, whether as working dogs or companions. We've taken them into our households and are responsible for fulfilling their basic and higher needs. For all the joy and companionship they give us, we owe our dog the following.

Adequate food and medical care

Exercise—not only the option for exercise but also the encouragement

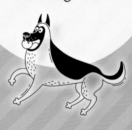

Grooming, ear and teeth cleaning, nail trimming, skin and coat conditioning

A life that is beyond mere survival

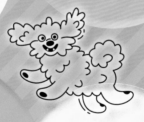

Exposure to the world beyond your fence

Twenty minutes each day of your undivided attention

Three enrichment activities per day (a walk, game of fetch, car ride)

Socialization with people and dogs outside your family

The right to give and receive unconditional love

Training, so your dog does not become a prisoner of their own misbehavior

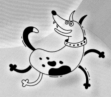

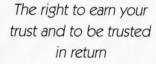

Fresh air and green grass

Respect for your dog's needs and wants

Responsible breeding, or none at all

Time and space all their own

The freedom to be foolish and silly and to make you laugh

The right to earn your trust and to be trusted in return

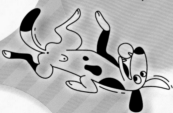

Forgiveness

The right to die with dignity

The honor of being remembered well

Operant Conditioning: The Motivation Quadrants

There are four ways to motivate an animal. We can **give** them something or **take** away something, in order to get them to **do** something or **stop doing** something.

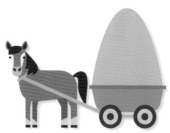

In the familiar cliché, there are two ways to get a cart horse to pull: lure them forward with a **carrot** or smack them from behind with a **stick**. In the first scenario, with the carrot, the horse is moved by a desire for a reward. In the second scenario, with the stick, they are moved by a desire to avoid pain. There are compelling reasons why we choose the carrot over the stick, not the least of which is because we choose to live and train joyfully.

POSITIVE REINFORCEMENT

When the dog does something good, give the dog a reward

NEGATIVE REINFORCEMENT

When the dog does something good, take away an aversive or boundary

POSITIVE PUNISHMENT

When the dog does something naughty, give the dog an aversive

NEGATIVE PUNISHMENT

When the dog does something naughty, take away a reward or privilege

Positive Reinforcement

Positive reinforcement training is a reward-based method in which the dog participates eagerly and joyfully.

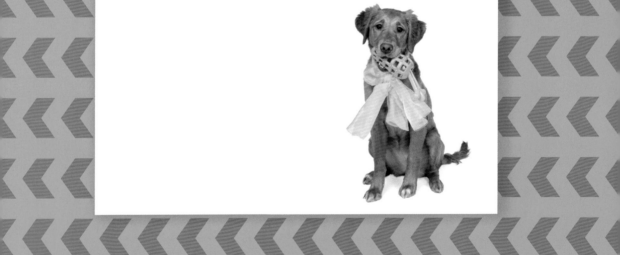

Positive reinforcement is the carrot in our cart-horse analogy. It means that we offer a reward for a behavior and allow it to be our dog's choice whether or not to do the behavior and get the reward. We don't force them, and we don't punish them.

This initially might sound like a flawed system, as we are leaving so much choice to the dog. In reality, however, it's an extremely effective method—much more effective than the "stick"—at motivating a dog and instilling in them a desire to please. The "carrot" leads to faster learning and higher retention of behavior.

Positive reinforcement training methods strengthen and enhance the relationship between you and your dog as you work collaboratively toward a mutual goal in an encouraging, stress-free, and fear-free environment. The dog participates in the learning process with a joyful attitude and enjoys interacting with the trainer.

A reward can come in different forms: a food treat, a toy, play, or praise and affection. When teaching a new behavior, food is most often used because it is high value and easy to dispense.

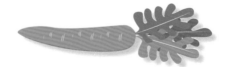

"Whatever needs to be maintained through force is doomed." —Henry Miller

Let's practice this lesson by teaching:

Which Hand Holds
the Treat?

We will practice the lesson of **positive reinforcement** by teaching our dog this simple trick. We hide a treat in one of our fists, then ask our dog to sniff each and indicate which hand holds the treat.

The positive reinforcement method means that when our dog picks correctly, they get rewarded. There is no punishment for choosing incorrectly; they simply get no reward. Your dog will be much more eager to play this game when they are not worried about being scolded.

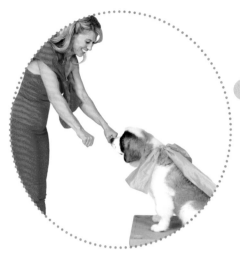

1 PRESENT BOTH FISTS

Hide a treat in one hand and encourage your dog to sniff both fists by saying, "Which hand?" Some dogs will indicate the correct hand with just a sensitive sniff, while other dogs will be more forceful.

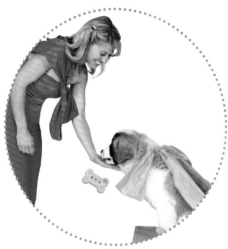

2 IF THEY ARE CORRECT

When your dog shows interest in the correct hand, say your **reward marker** word and open your hand. That's **positive reinforcement**!

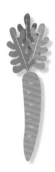

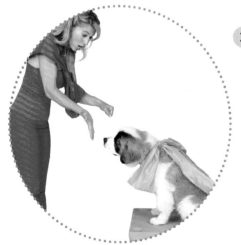

3 IF THEY ARE INCORRECT

Did your indicate the wrong hand? Open it and show them the empty hand. You can say, "Whoops! Try again," but avoid saying, "No" or scolding them. Try it again.

Train Joyfully!

You want your dog to be motivated to train, looking forward to it as a highlight of their day. Every bit of enthusiasm that you inject into your training session will speed up your dog's learning. Follow these simple tips to keep your dog (and yourself!) joyfully motivated.

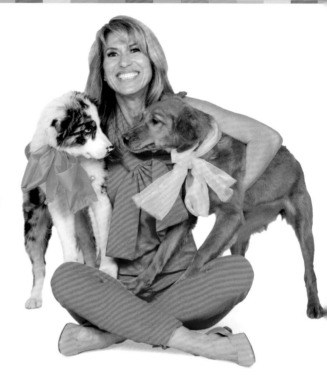

USE YOUR HAPPY VOICE

When your dog does something right, use your high-pitched "happy voice," which is instinctively rewarding. Your happy voice should rise in pitch at the end in a sing-songy tone.

LEAVE THEM WANTING MORE

End your training session while everyone is having a good time and before your dog gets tired or bored. Quit with them wanting more so they look forward to the next session.

END ON A HIGH NOTE

Keep your dog's confidence up by always ending your training session on a successful note, even if you have to go back to an easier behavior to achieve this. Ask your dog for a behavior they know well, praise them excitedly for it, and end the session then.

BLUR THE LINE BETWEEN PLAY AND WORK

If you're not having fun during your training session, then your dog is probably not either. Don't plod through an uninspiring training session or your dog will associate training, and you, with boredom. Motivate your dog! Blur the line between play and work. Incorporate a toy reward after a great effort, and play a few minutes after every training session.

BE A FUN PERSON TO BE AROUND!

The more fun you are, the more your dog will value your attention, and the more motivated they will be to please you. Make life fun and exciting in your presence! Give treats, throw balls, make funny noises, laugh, and smile.

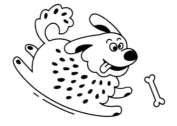

Enthusiasm and positivity make life worth living.

Reward Success;
Ignore the Rest

In positive reinforcement training, we reward our dog for getting it right and ignore unsuccessful attempts without punishing them.

A dog doesn't learn anything when they get something wrong. A dog learns when they get it right—and they get rewarded.

During the learning process we need our dog to problem solve through experimentation. We need them to try a lot of different behaviors so that we can let them know (with a reward marker or treat) which ones were correct. That skill of trying lots of different things is called **offering behaviors** and is incredibly useful in training.

If we were to say "No" every time our dog offered a behavior that didn't happen to be correct, they would become reluctant to try anything at all. They'd rather do nothing than be wrong. Which is why we **reward success** and simply **ignore the rest**.

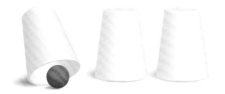

Happiness is to be needed and wanted by those we love.

Let's practice this lesson by teaching:

Cup and Ball Game

Let's teach our dog a classic game in which we ask them to find the ball hidden beneath one of three cups. We'll put a canine twist on it, however, and use a meatball instead of a ball and plant pots that have convenient "scent holes" at the top.

Dogs can be very sensitive about being wrong. If your dog indicates an incorrect pot, don't say "No," but rather encourage them to keep looking. **Reward success** and **ignore the rest.**

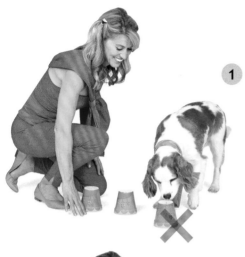

1 PRESENT THE CHALLENGE

Hide a meatball under one cup. Encourage your dog to sniff all three by tapping each one. If they are on the wrong cup, **ignore it** or encourage them to "Keep looking!"

2 BE OBSERVANT

Dogs will vary in how they indicate the correct cup. In the beginning they usually give only a soft, short sniff. Be observant and notice that subtle indication.

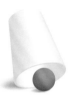

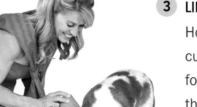

3 LIFT THE CUP

Hooray! **Reward success** by lifting the cup. In this game it is even more fun for your dog to get the treat from under the cup, where they discovered it, than to get it from your hand.

Learning Occurs with Successes

A dog only learns when they get it right—and get rewarded. Set low enough criteria that your dog can get many successful attempts.

A dog learns when they get it right and they get rewarded. Every time a treat gets popped into their mouth, it strengthens a connection in their brain. The more successful repetitions they have, the faster they learn.

If you set a training goal that is too ambitious, and your dog is never successful and never gets a treat, then your dog learns nothing. **Learning only occurs with successful attempts.**

In order to get as many successful attempts as possible, we want to make it easy for our dog to do the behavior correctly. If you are teaching them to fetch, have them fetch an object that is only a few feet away, and reward that. And reward it again, and again.

If you make the challenge too difficult for your dog or require too much, you won't have as many opportunities to reward, and that brain pathway won't be built as quickly.

Don't set up your dog for a task that is beyond their capabilities or knowledge, as it is a prescription for failure. Instead, lower the **criteria for success** and coach them toward this goal. Help them get it right and reward them excitedly for their success!

A dog learns from successes, not failures.

Let's practice this lesson by teaching:

Take a Bow

When taking a bow, your dog's front elbows touch the floor. To keep your dog from lying down, we will employ the **modeling** technique and use a Magic Square to help compel the behavior.

At first, your dog's elbows may only dip slightly but not far enough to touch the floor. We will reward just that. We will set low enough criteria so that the dog can get many successful attempts because **learning occurs with successes**.

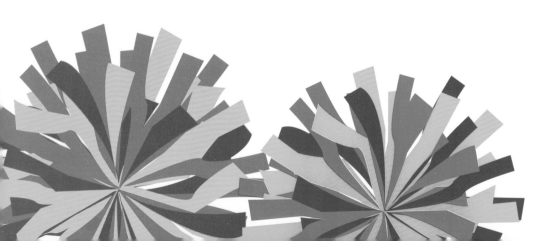

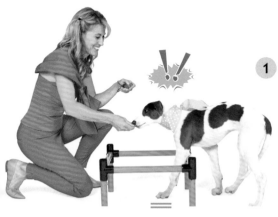

1 LURE YOUR DOG INTO THE SQUARE

Use a treat to lure your dog into the square. **Click** and **treat** this small success.

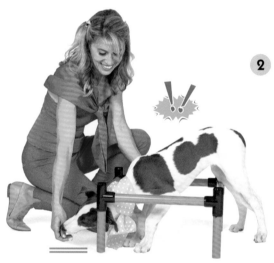

2 REWARD SMALL SUCCESSES

We will not require our dog to go all the way down into a bow just yet. Instead, we will **repeatedly reward** them for whatever stage they can give us easily, such as a partial elbow dip.

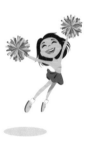

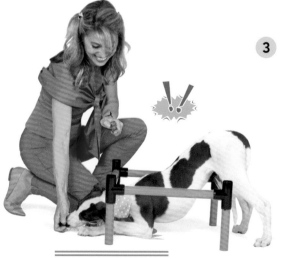

3 PROGRESS AND RAISE THE CRITERIA

Once your dog is able to easily and repeatedly get the previous step, raise the criteria and require a little more of them. If your dog is not getting a success within about twenty seconds, **regress** to the previous criteria.

Let's practice this lesson by teaching:

Retrieve an Object

Some dogs are natural retrievers. Other dogs have to be taught, incrementally, to fetch an object. We will use the "pan retrieve" method and get **many successful repetitions** of small retrieves.

We hand the dog a toy, and they will probably immediately drop it where it will fall into a pan below, making a clanging sound. The clang is the **reward marker**, just like a clicker would be. Every time we hear a clang, our dog gets a treat.

Then we **progress** and raise the criteria. We move the pan slightly to the side. The dog will have to consciously move their head to drop the toy into the pan. Eventually we will throw the toy across the room and have them bring it back to the pan.

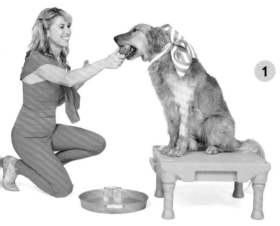

1 HAND YOUR DOG A TOY

Set a metal pan in front of your dog—it helps if they are on a raised surface. Hand them a toy they will willingly open their mouth for, such as a treat-filled toy. Use a toy that is hard enough to make a sound when it hits the pan.

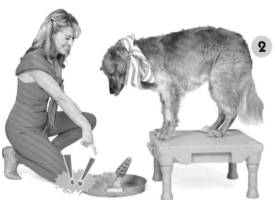

2 GET THEM TO DROP IT IN THE PAN

A dog will usually drop the toy within a few seconds. (If yours doesn't, use a lower-value toy.) The toy will fall into the pan. When you hear the *clang,* give your dog a treat!

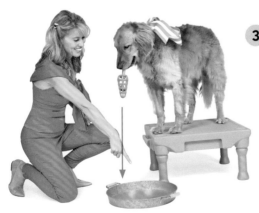

3 MOVE THE PAN TO THE SIDE

After many successful drops, move the pan slightly. If your dog misses the pan, say a lighthearted "Whoops!" and hand them the toy again. If they miss three times in a row, **regress** to the previous step.

Jackpot Rewards

Increase motivation by giving your dog a jackpot—a whole handful of treats—when they perform exceptionally well.

We know the lure of a jackpot—having achieved it once, we will sit at the slot machine all night in hopes of being rewarded again with that elusive prize. We can also use a **jackpot reward** to motivate our dog.

Ask your dog to perform some tricks that they are working on. If they do them fairly well, give them a small reward. If they perform the behavior very well, or better than they have in the past, *jackpot* . . . give them a whole handful of treats! That wil make an impression on them. They will continue trying extra hard in hopes of hitting that jackpot again.

Using several different types of treats during a training session can also keep your dog motivated—a goldfish cracker for a mediocre effort and a hot dog for a good effort, for example.

A session of tug, if your dog enjoys that, is another great jackpot reward. Keep the tug toy in your back pocket and whip it out when your dog does something really great!

Reward moments, not only complete behaviors.

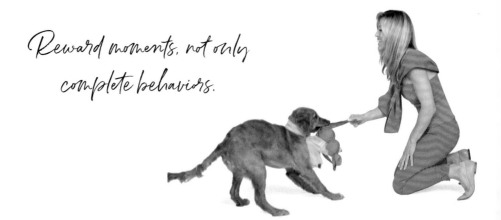

Breed Motivation

Breed characteristics influence a dog's primary motivations. Knowledge of your dog's breed can help you tailor your training program to take advantage of their unique skills.

Herding dogs are people-focused and take instruction readily. They are quick learners who are prey driven and often value a flying disc reward over food.

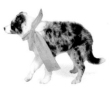

BORDER COLLIE

Working dogs were bred to perform a specific job, such as guarding property, pulling sleds, or performing rescues. They are large and strong and can be assertive, stubborn, and independent.

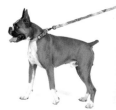

BOXER

Sporting dogs were bred to find by scent and retrieve prey for their hunting masters (notice their long noses), and they enjoy scent games. Sporting dogs are athletic and very food motivated.

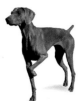

WEIMARANER

Hounds are hunters; some track with their nose (bloodhounds) while others chase moving things by sight (greyhounds). Hounds can be easily distracted, so it's best to train in an empty environment.

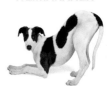

GREYHOUND

Terriers are named after Terra (earth), as most were designed to hunt vermin in the ground. Terriers are feisty and energetic, and they love a reward of a game of tug, as it imitates the shaking of a vermin.

TERRIER

Toy breeds were bred as companions. They are small and quick, so your timing must be spot-on. Everything they do must be their choice.

CHIHUAHUA

Nonfood Rewards

Food is a reward, but it's not the only one. A toy, attention, praise, play, and access to areas and resources are all rewards too.

Treats are a powerful reward, but there are other rewards we can give to our dog as well. By incorporating **nonfood rewards** into our training, we gain more options for rewarding our dog.

Dogs with a high prey drive will work for rewards of a flying disc, ball, or game of tug. A toy reward can be used in conjunction with food: you can routinely reward your dog from your treat bag and then **jackpot** them with the toy when they do something especially great. Or you can throw a flying disc as a reward, and when your dog brings it back, trade them the disc for a treat. That makes the disc even more valuable!

Access to resources and areas is also a reward. These resources can include food, toys, your bed, and the outdoors. On the next page we will have your dog perform a behavior that is rewarded with outdoor access.

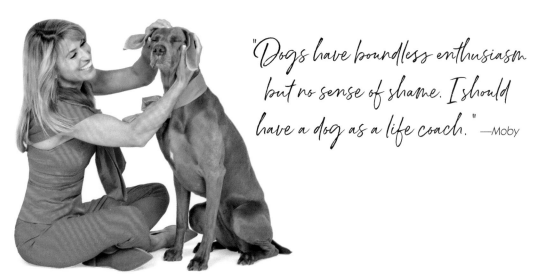

"Dogs have boundless enthusiasm but no sense of shame. I should have a dog as a life coach." —Moby

Let's practice this lesson by teaching:

Ring a Bell to Go Out

We will teach your dog to ring a bell hanging from the doorknob when they want to go out. This is a great tool in potty training, and even very young puppies can easily learn the skill. During initial training we will use food as a reward, but once the dog has learned the behavior we will switch to the **nonfood reward** of access to the outdoors.

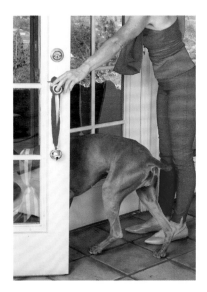

Access to the outdoors is a reward.

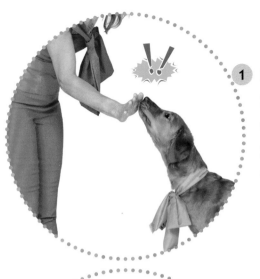

1 NOSE-TOUCH YOUR HAND

Hold out one hand and hold your **clicker** and a **treat** in the other. When your dog touches your hand, click your clicker and follow up with a treat.

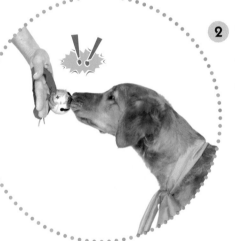

2 WRAP THE BELL AROUND YOUR HAND

Say, "Bell" and hold out your hand. Again, click and treat.

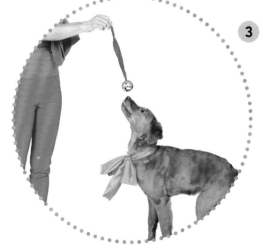

3 DANGLE THE BELL

Your dog will want to nose-touch your hand, so hold the bell high over their head so that they are only able to reach the bell portion and not your hand. Reward success by opening the door for them.

Self-Control

TECHNIQUES TO TURN OFF FRUSTRATION

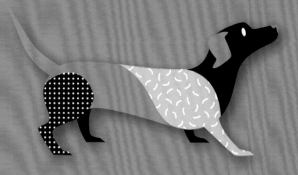

Part of dog training is getting a dog excited and interested in learning. Another part of dog training is getting a dog to calm down and focus.

Dogs do not naturally practice **self-control**. They act on impulses such as charging the front door, pulling on their leash, snatching food from your hands or the counter, jumping on people, and chasing cats.

In this chapter we will learn techniques to teach our dog to control their **impulses**. We'll use positive methods that offer rewards for self-control and outlets to **redirect** our dog's energy into positive pursuits. Our dog will learn rules of proper conduct and willingly abide by them in order to get what they want.

Having a clear strategy for dealing with unwanted behavior from your dog will alleviate frustration for both you and your dog.

"Once you have had a wonderful dog, a life without one is a life diminished."
—Dean Koontz

Impulse Control

Dogs are impulsive. But we can teach them that by practicing self-control, they can actually get what they want—or at least get another reward.

With dogs as with children, we want to teach them that they need to give in order to get. They need to say "Please" before they get a reward. Having this respectful relationship allows our dog to be a true family member. **Self-control** is like a muscle that gets stronger with repeated use. Small demonstrations of politeness every day build your dog's capacity for self-control.

Some ways to practice giving in order to get include having your dog sit before receiving their meal, having them stand still to get leashed up for a walk, or having them drop their ball before you'll throw it again.

We will teach our dog to have patience and **impulse control** using all positive methods. We will not scold our dog but rather will leave the choice up to them and allow them figure out on their own that the best rewards come to those who practice self-control.

Self-control is choosing what you want most over what you want now.

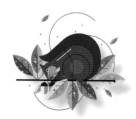

Let's practice this lesson by teaching:

Loose-Leash Walking

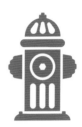

In this lesson we will tackle one of the most frustrating **impulse control** challenges: teaching our dog to not pull and to walk on a loose leash.

Traditionally this has been taught with aversion methods—namely, jerking the leash. With most dogs, this is not a lasting solution (nor is is pleasant for you or for your dog). Instead, we will get our dog to **choose** to slacken the leash out of their own free will. Here is how we are going to do it.

Let's say your dog is out for a walk and sees a fire hydrant that they really want to investigate. They pull on the leash. You are goint to stop walking. You are going to stand still until the leash slackens. Only with a slack leash will your dog be allowed to walk to the hydrant. Your dog will never get to where they want with a taut leash. Without being forced, your dog will **choose** to slacken the leash.

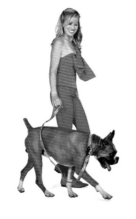

1 START YOUR WALK

Start walking. Keep walking so long as the leash is slack (which may only be a few seconds).

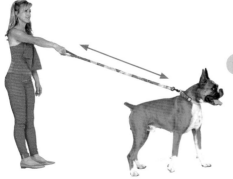

2 WHEN YOUR DOG PULLS, STOP

Don't say "No." Merely plant your feet. Your dog is prevented from getting to where they want. We **reward success and ignore the rest**.

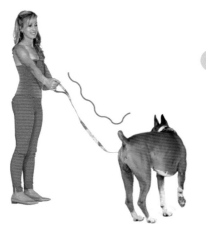

3 WAIT FOR THE LEASH TO SLACKEN

After a while, your dog will turn back to you and slacken the leash. You can also pat your leg and call to them to get them to turn back.

4 WALK WHERE THEY WANT

With a slack leash, walk where your dog wants to go. They will learn that they never get to their goal with a taut leash, only with a slack leash.

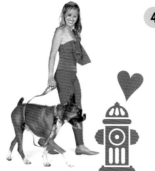

Extinction

A dog will repeat a behavior that you have been rewarding. If you want that behavior to stop, stop rewarding it. This will result in behavior extinction.

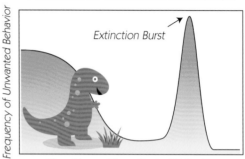

PROCESS OF BEHAVIOR EXTINCTION

Frequency of Unwanted Behavior

Extinction Burst

Time Elapsed from Start of Extinction

We may have inadvertently caused our dog to develop some bad habits. Perhaps we gave them a few table scraps over the years, and now they beg incessantly throughout our dinner. We want this behavior to stop. So . . . we stop rewarding it. We go through an **extinction** process. If we stop giving our dog scraps from the table, they will eventually stop begging at the table.

To extinguish an unwanted behavior, you need not do anything more than refrain from rewarding it. During the process of extinction, the unwanted behavior will often get worse before it gets better, in a flurry of attempts known as an **extinction burst**. The dog will not immediately give up the behavior once they have stopped being rewarded for it but rather try the behavior again and again, harder, faster, more emphatically, in a burst of activity.

This extinction burst usually occurs right before the dog finally gives up. Hang in there! If at all possible, ignore your dog's misbehavior during this extinction burst, as giving attention to it will likely cause the behavior to get even worse.

We achieve success through perseverance, not strength.

Positive Redirection

Instead of scolding, we redirect misbehavior into a more positive pursuit. We redirect an action, substitute an object, and reward the new behavior.

We want to stop unwanted behavior before it becomes a habit. Intervene early; redirect your dog before they're invested in whatever havoc they're about to wreak. With positive redirection, we **redirect** our dog to do something else, we **substitute** the object they are playing with, and then we **reward** them for doing the right thing. To redirect your dog, simply call their name in a happy voice. When they look at you, give them something else to do or chew on. Great work—you stopped a habit before it got a chance to put down roots.

If you catch your dog chewing on your shoe, take it from them and substitute with an appropriate chew toy.

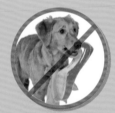

CHEW YOUR SHOE   **CHEW A BONE**

If your dog barks, redirect by asking them to lie down (dogs don't usually bark when lying down) and reward them for doing so.

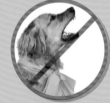

BARK   **LIE DOWN**

If your dog dashes out the door, redirect by asking them to go to their home base (see page 122) and reward them there.

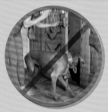
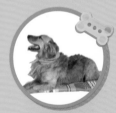
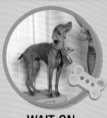

DOOR DASH   **WAIT ON HOME BASE**

Home Base

A raised platform acts as a "home base" for your dog, giving them a default, secure spot. This quiets your dog and helps manage their movement.

When we're eating dinner, we can have our dog lie calmly on their home base. Rather than bolting when we open the front door, our dog can wait momentarily on their home base. When we are trying to give instruction to our distracted dog, we can get their attention by confining their busy feet to a home base ("Quiet feet equal a focused mind").

A **home base** is a small, raised platform. It needs to be small enough that it quiets your dog's busy feet and high enough that it takes some effort to get off of it. Dogs are naturally height-seeking, and they enjoy being on a raised platform because it makes them feel more in charge (think of puppies playing King of the Hill). Increase the value of the home base by using it to give routine rewards; have your dog wait on their home base before getting their dinner and go to their home base to get pet. If you make the platform a rewarding place to be (with treats and petting), your dog will take to it very quickly, and you'll likely find them jumping on it without having been asked!

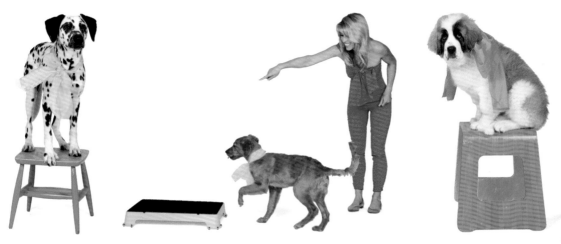

Let's practice this lesson by teaching:

Send/Stay on Platform

With **home-base training** you will be able to send your dog to the platform from anywhere in the room and have your dog stay on the platform until released. Here are some tips to help train these goals:

- Reward your dog for getting *on* the platform, but never reward them for getting *off* the platform. We don't want them randomly jumping off because they think they will get a reward.

- Don't allow your dog to get off of the platform at will. Only allow them off at your direction.

- If they *do* get off by their own decision, direct them back on again.

- If your dog is staying on the platform, periodically give them a treat up there.

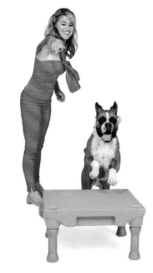

1 SEND TO HOME BASE

In lesson 5 we taught our dog to **go to a mark**. Let's build on that skill and send our dog to the raised platform. Always reward in the **correct position**: on the platform.

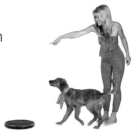

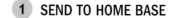

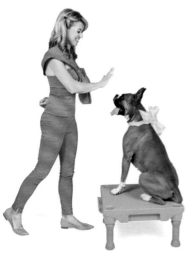

2 STAY ON HOME BASE

In lesson 10 we taught our dog to **stay in a square**. Let's progress to teach them to stay on their home base.

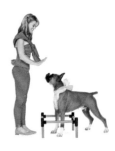

3 INCREASE DISTANCE, DURATION, AND DISTRACTIONS

Practice circling the platform, holding the stay for longer, and introducing distractions. Anticipate your dog breaking their stay and stop it by firmly saying "Stay," moving toward them, and making eye contact.

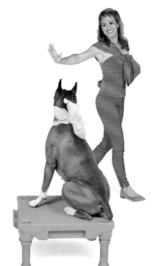

"Now and then it's good to pause in our pursuit of happiness and just be happy."
—Guillaume Apollinaire

People are their most beautiful when they follow their passions.

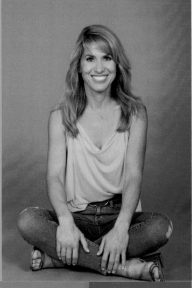

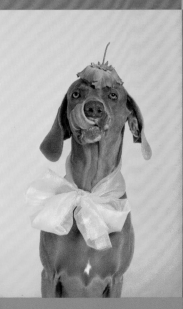

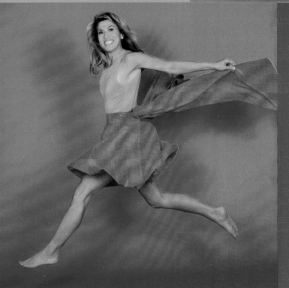

Wake up anticipating something great is going to happen today!

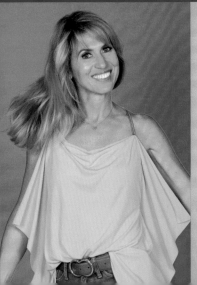

Be your own kind of beautiful.

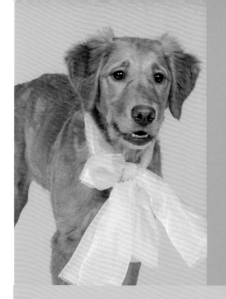

Enthusiasm is the electricity of life. We only become old if we lose that spark.

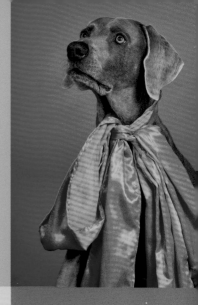

"If you have good thoughts they will shine out of your face like sunbeams and you will always look lovely." —Roald Dahl

Always find time for the things that make you feel happy to be alive.

"I suppose if we couldn't laugh at things that don't make sense, we couldn't react to a lot of life."
—Bill Watterson

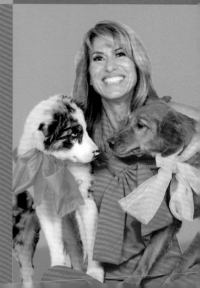

Enrichment

THE SIX COMPONENTS OF JOY

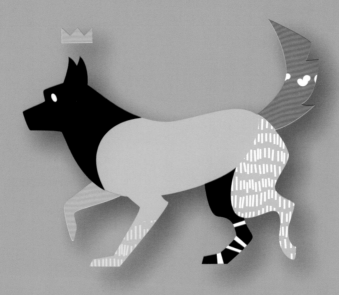

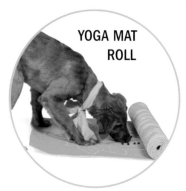

YOGA MAT
ROLL

Dogs don't want to lie on the couch all day. They want to be challenged and excited and puzzled; they want to learn new things and have you congratulate them on their discoveries! Try these busy challenges with your dog.

YOGA MAT ROLL Lay your yoga mat flat and sprinkle treats on it. Roll it up. Encourage your dog to use their nose to unroll it. Each nose shove should reveal a treat, so it becomes a self-rewarding game.

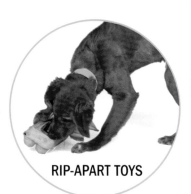

RIP-APART TOYS

RIP-APART TOYS Rather than having your expensive dog toys ripped up, give your dog some designated rip-apart toys, such as paper egg cartons, paper-towel rolls, and cardboard boxes.

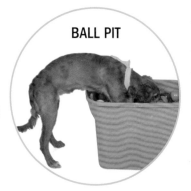

BALL PIT

BALL PIT Hide a dog biscuit in a ball pit, and let your dog search it out. In lieu of balls, use a box of packing material or crumpled newspaper balls.

MUFFIN TIN Put treats in the cups of a muffin tin and cover each treat with a tennis ball. Let your dog puzzle over how to get the treats.

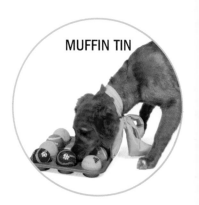

MUFFIN TIN

Puzzle Challenges

Puzzles challenge your dog's mind to solve a novel problem. They offer an opportunity for your dog to feel the joy of success!

A dog will find more joy in searching out kibble piece by piece than in being handed it in a convenient bowl. **Puzzle challenges** are all around us, and once you devise a few, you will see puzzle opportunities hiding in all sorts of common household items: cardboard boxes, egg cartons, paper tubes, and more. Here are a few puzzles to get you and your dog started.

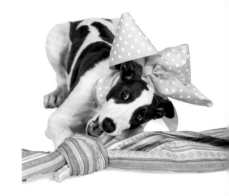

BONE IN A TOWEL Tie a rawhide bone or several treats in a knotted towel. Let your dog struggle to get them out.

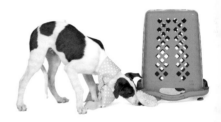

TOY UNDER A BASKET Hide your dog's favorite toy, or a food-filled toy, under a laundry basket. They can see it and smell it, but how can they get it?

BLANKET TOSS Toss a blanket over your dog and encourage them to struggle out of it. Toss the blanket over yourself. Where did you go?

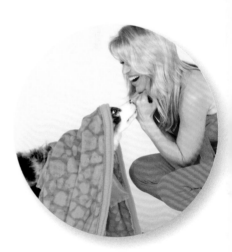

"Willingness to be puzzled is a valuable trait to cultivate, from childhood to advanced inquiry." —Noam Chomsky

Exploration

Build your dog's confidence by encouraging them to explore novel situations. Successful exploration will alleviate fears and bring joy to your dog.

A key to overcoming fear is being allowed to approach the feared object at your own pace and to have it result in good (or at least not bad) things. Never push your dog toward a feared object; allow them an escape and control the outcome. If you know a loud bang will scare your dog, mitigate that threat by doing something to muffle the sound.

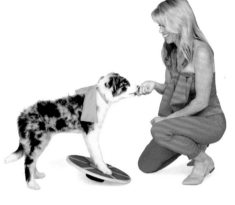

WOBBLE BOARD A tool in canine conditioning, this disc has a half-dome fulcrum, which lets it wobble in every direction. Use treats to entice your dog to explore this strange object.

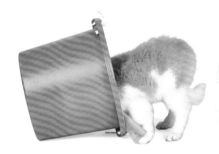

FIND THE HIDDEN TREATS Hide kibble, goldfish crackers, or cereal pieces all over the house: under chairs, inside toys, and behind pillows. Start with a few out in the open to get your dog going.

TUNNEL Start with the tunnel scrunched up short. Place treats inside and encourage your dog to explore.

HIDE AND SEEK Hide behind a door and call happily to your dog. Have treats ready when they find you.

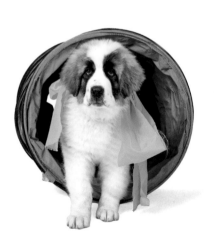

Choice

Find opportunities to allow your dog choices. This helps them feel like they have some power and control over what they do, and it also provides an opportunity for communication.

Our dogs are mostly told what to do; we decide where we are going and what we are doing and when we play and how we play. So it's nice to find opportunities for our dog to have a **choice**. Shall we go down the left path or the right path? Do you prefer cheese or chicken for a treat? Do you want to play flying disc or ball?

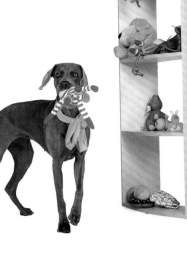

Where does your dog prefer to sleep? Move their dog bed for a few nights and see whether they indicate a preference (such as by lying on the floor in the spot where their bed used to be). Does your dog want to be outside? Teaching them to use a doggy doorbell (lesson 20) allows them to communicate their desire.

Does your dog have dozens of toys accessible? After the initial excitement of a new toy, does it lie unnoticed in the toy box? Give your dog decision-making joy by letting them chose a "toy of the day." Put away all of their toys on a shelf. Once a day, take your dog to the shelf and allow them to pick out just one to play with. Interestingly, dogs seem to get more joy out of this one toy than the dozens they had before.

"*A beautiful day begins with a beautiful mindset.*" —*John Geiger*

Desire to Be Loved

Your dog thinks about you more than any other thing in their life. Show you love them by giving them your kind attention, touch, and words.

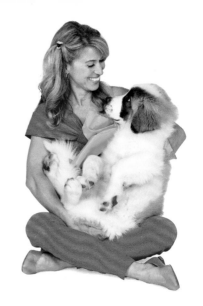

Just as we know when our dogs love us, they know when we love them. They see it in our eyes and hear it in our joyful voice. They understand our apology when we trip over them, and they submit to our gentle care when cleaning their ears, clipping their nails, or treating a wound. They allow themselves to be dressed in a coat without resentment, as they trust in our love and understand our good intentions.

Dogs are happy with what they get, so it can be all too easy to put aside their needs in favor of "more important" things, such as work, housecleaning, and social obligations. Here are some ways we can tell our dog we love them:

- Gaze softly into their eyes—dogs communicate with each other through eye contact, so they will instinctively understand your intention
- Rub their ears—what a joy!
- Snuggle or sleep together
- Lean on your dog (like they sometimes do to you)
- Talk to your dog
- Watch them, give them attention, and congratulate them on chasing the lizard, digging the hole, or finding the treasure

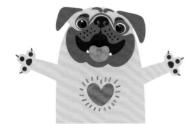

There is only one happiness in life; to love and be loved.

Order

Dogs are pack animals that have an instinct to live in a structured environment with order and rules. Order gives dogs predictability and alleviates fears of being abandoned or not being fed.

Structure is security and predictability. It allows dogs to live without the constant stress of not knowing when dinner is coming or wondering whether they have been abandoned every time you leave the room. Dogs take comfort in routine. They are easily pattern trained and enjoy the small rituals built into their daily lives.

What are some ways we can build predictability and ritual into our routine? We can have our dog sit before receiving their dinner. A bedtime ritual can be as simple as a kiss on the head. When you leave the house, have a special way of letting your dog know you are leaving so they don't worry you have left the house every time you leave the room. Dogs are extremely good associative learners, so they are quick to learn that picking up your keys means you are leaving and putting on your sneakers means that you are taking them for a walk. These little rituals will come to be a special bond between the two of you—a secret language all your own.

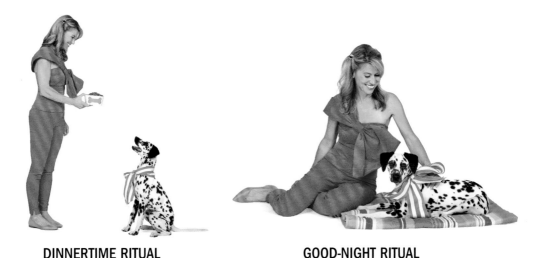

DINNERTIME RITUAL   **GOOD-NIGHT RITUAL**

Sense of Humor and Play

Nothing makes a dog happier than a loving and playful owner. Dogs enjoy playing jokes on us, and they enjoy having gentle jokes played upon them as well.

Dogs enjoy **play** and understand **humor**.
Try a magic trick with your dog: stand
in a doorway looking at your dog, raise
a blanket above your head so as to fully
conceal yourself, and when you drop the
blanket, poof! You've vanished behind the
wall. Where did you go?! Play with your dog's
ball and make it magically disappear into your
back pocket. The moment of puzzlement for your dog is
rewarded with ecstatic joy upon finding the missing person or toy.

Dogs will play tricks on you as well! Your dog may lay their stick on
the ground and feign disinterest until you reach for it, then at the
last moment snatch it and dart away! Your dog may grab a shoe
and goad you into chasing them. And you might be lucky enough to
see your dog laugh and prance in sheer joy.

Play is enthusiasm for life!

Congratulations! By finishing this book, you've demonstrated a commitment to your dog's well-being through enriching their life with joyful training and challenges. You've shown a commitment to the close bonded relationship the two of you share. You've come a long way! Even if you haven't reached all of your goals yet, recognize that change is an ongoing process. Take a moment to acknowledge your accomplishments.

THROUGH THIS BOOK, I HAVE:

- [ ] Impressed my friends with new dog tricks
- [ ] Challenged my dog's brain
- [ ] Increased my skill as a dog trainer
- [ ] Bonded with my dog
- [ ] Taught my dog to be better behaved
- [ ] Increased my dog's confidence and self-esteem
- [ ] Taught my dog useful behaviors
- [ ] Discovered outlets for my dog's energy
- [ ] Showed my dog that I love them
- [ ] Become more joyful
- [ ] Learned correct and humane training methods
- [ ] Discovered more about my dog
- [ ] Other: _____

*Whether they're young or old, athletic or lazy, quick-witted or dumb as a rock, they're your dog, and their success need only be measured in your eyes. I hope this book inspires you to **Do More with Your Dog!***

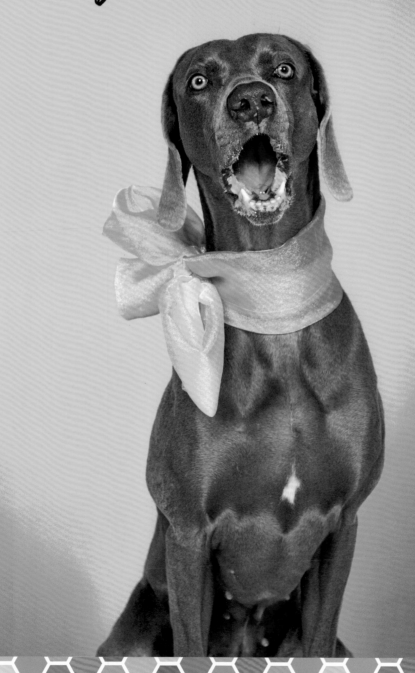

You did it!

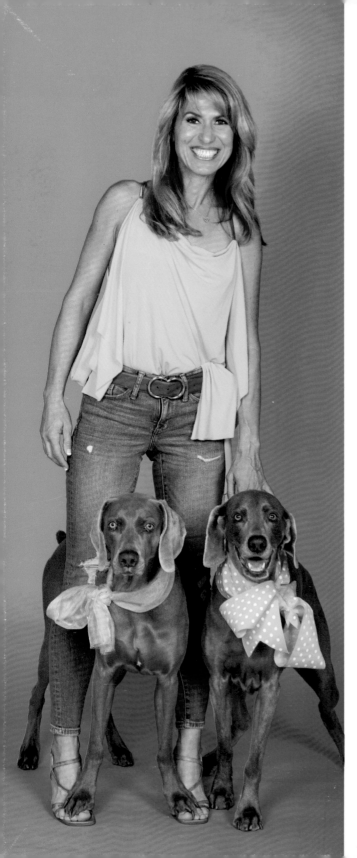

KYRA SUNDANCE is a world-renowned dog trainer, lecturer, and internationally best-selling author. With over a million copies in print, Kyra's award-winning books, kits, and videos have inspired dog owners worldwide to develop fun and rewarding relationships with their dogs.

Honed through decades of professional experience, Kyra's easy-to-follow instructions are the most effective and humane way to train, using positive methods that foster confident, happy dogs.

Kyra is a professional set trainer for movie dogs and a professional stunt dog performer starring in shows for the king of Morocco, Disney's Hollywood stage shows, circuses, NBA halftime shows, *The Tonight Show, The Ellen DeGeneres Show*, and numerous other TV shows and movies.

As Chief Joy Officer of Do More With Your Dog!, Kyra presents widely popular workshops and online certification courses on dog tricks, training, and canine fitness.

Kyra is nationally ranked in competitive dog sports and an avid ultrarunner.

Jadie and Kimba live with Kyra at their ranch in California's Mojave Desert.

DoMoreWithYourDog.com